THE STRUGGLE YOU CAN'T SEE

The Struggle You Can't See

Experiences of Neurodivergent and Invisibly
Disabled Students in Higher Education

Ash Lierman

OpenBook
Publishers

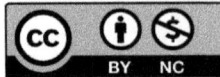

https://www.openbookpublishers.com

©2024 Ash Lierman

ISBN Paperback: 978-1-80511-374-4
ISBN Hardback: 978-1-80511-375-1
ISBN Digital (PDF): 978-1-80511-376-8
ISBN Digital eBook (EPUB): 978-1-80511-377-5
ISBN HTML: 978-1-80511-378-2

DOI: 10.11647/OBP.0420

Cover image: A stack of books with a ladder leaning against it, September 23, 2023, Unsplash+ in collaboration with 8machine, licensed under the Unsplash+ License, https://unsplash.com/photos/a-stack-of-books-with-a-ladder-leaning-against-it-KIqVxfgwx-w
Cover design: Jeevanjot Kaur Nagpal

Contents

About the Author

Dr. Ash Lierman (they/them) is the Instruction & Education Librarian at Campbell Library on the Glassboro campus of Rowan University, in southern New Jersey, USA. They are also the chair of Rowan University Libraries' DEI Committee. They support teaching and learning across the university, particularly for the College of Education, graduate students, and online learners. As a disabled, queer, nonbinary and agender librarian, their research and professional interests focus on social justice for marginalized academic library users and workers, especially those who are disabled and LGBTQ+. They have also co-contributed a chapter to *Toward Inclusive Academic Librarian Hiring Practices* (Houk, Nielsen, & Wong-Welch, eds.), published in 2024 by the Association of College and Research Libraries (ACRL).

List of Abbreviations

ACE	American Council on Education
ADA	Americans with Disabilities Act (USA)
ADAAA	Americans with Disabilities Act Amendments Act (USA)
ADHD	Attention deficit hyperactivity disorder
AHEAD	Association on Higher Education and Disability (USA)
BPD	Bipolar disorder
CAST	Center for Applied Special Technology
CIL	Centers for Independent Living
DCC	Disability cultural center
DEI	Diversity, equity and inclusion
DisCrit	Disability critical race theory
DSE	Disability studies in education
GAD	Generalized anxiety disorder
GPA	Grade point average
IDEA	Individuals with Disabilities Education Act (USA)
IEP	Individualized education plan
LGBTQ+	Lesbian, gay, bisexual/pansexual, transgender, queer/questioning, and other related identities
ME	Myalgic encephalomyelitis (also known as chronic fatigue syndrome)
NCES	National Center for Education Statistics (USA)
NTACT	National Technical Assistance Center on Transition (USA)

OCD   Obsessive-compulsive disorder

PDSP   Physically Disabled Students' Program (Berkeley University)

PTSD   Post-traumatic stress disorder

STEM   Science, technology, engineering, and mathematics

TBI   Traumatic brain injury/injuries

UC   University of California

UDL   Universal Design for Learning

Introduction

Purpose, Approach, and Guiding Principles

At this point in my early forties, I have quite literally lost count of the number of my friends and colleagues who have been diagnosed with life-altering abbreviations: ADHD, BPD, ME, GAD, and more. Almost universally, at least in my personal sphere of experience, these diagnoses were also made not in their childhood, but far later. The string of letters that changed everything only appeared in their lives at thirty, at thirty-five, at forty—but in retrospect, it became an explanation that brought on a torrent of emotional relief, regret, and belated understanding. Some of these people I had known for long enough to share that torrent. I was able to recall vivid memories of a younger friend breaking down in tears on the sofa in my apartment, for example, as she tried to force herself to complete an assignment for a college class with my wife and me present for accountability, but still failed to even begin. I remember being bewildered, at the time, as to what the problem could be, and why what seemed to me like a relatively simple task could be so impossible for her. Even so, though, in the face of her tears of frustration, I could not doubt that it was.

Even as hearing her diagnosis finally made sense of that memory, though, it also connected other uncomfortable dots in my mind. After all, I had received my own string of letters some time earlier, although still only when I was nearly thirty years old. Mine was OCD: which does not stand for someone's thoughtless joke about preferring order and cleanliness, but for diagnosed obsessive-compulsive disorder, and chronic depression along with it. As I reviewed my own experiences as a college student, I realized that although starting a paper had never been an insurmountable task for me personally, at times other things had

    https://doi.org/10.11647/OBP.0420.00

been that would have seemed equally simple to anyone else: sleeping through the night, getting out of bed in the morning to attend classes and examinations, joining conversations in class, and sharing a room with another person, to name a few. I had just assumed that, although these felt like impossibilities for no reason I could understand, it must actually only be laziness and weakness of moral character that made them feel that way, since so many adults in my life so far had already been at pains to tell me so. I have no doubt that my friend assumed the same in her case.

All the same, I genuinely believe that most of the educators who became frustrated with me as a child, adolescent, and young adult had my best interests at heart, and would have helped me if they had been able. Not every educator has personally experienced being a student trying to cope with seemingly impossible tasks, or has completely unpacked that experience even if they have. Even faculty and staff who work directly with students, for that matter, are not always in the position of being present at the moment when an aspect of a student's body or mind proves to be completely incompatible with rigid academic demands. My young friend's professors were not able to sit on the sofa beside her, witnessing with their own eyes that her failure was not for any lack of trying. When a student has unique needs that are not outwardly visible, there are few opportunities to see personally the evidence of just how real and severe their struggle is. The students themselves may not even realize that what they are experiencing is far more difficult than it should be.

If students are to succeed in higher education, in a way that is equally accessible and fair to all, it is imperative to reduce the number of experiences like those my friend and I had. Invisibly disabled and neurodivergent students should not have to go through higher education under disproportionate, isolating burdens, facing seemingly impossible demands that are treated like simple tasks, and not even understanding why. To accomplish this, however, the educators, families, and peers of those students will have to learn more about what we can't always see: which is what those students actually experience in college. In many cases, the students themselves need to be helped to see it better, too.

The Purpose of This Book

To this end, this book aims to compile existing research on neurodivergent and invisibly disabled students' experiences in higher education, mostly in English-speaking countries around the world, in a comprehensive and organized way. By this time, there is an extensive body of scholarly and professional literature available on this topic. Hundreds of studies have been published based on interviews with students individually or in groups, all sharing a single diagnosis or all facing different types of challenges, in which the students recount to an interviewer their experiences, barriers, supports, and suggestions for improvement in the college environment. What does not seem to have been attempted to date, however, is a truly broad analysis of the themes and patterns in this literature, which brings together multiple threads of similar types of experience and examines where they overlap, where they agree, and what they suggest. This book attempts to fill that gap, by identifying the things that invisibly disabled and neurodivergent students have already told us, in study after study, hurt and help them most in higher education.

This information will be of value, of course, to staff and faculty in higher education who work with students of all kinds, and want to know what they and their institutions can do to better serve this specific population. It will also, however, be of value for anyone who is interested in learning what these students experience in college, and, as mentioned above, that includes invisibly disabled and neurodivergent students themselves. 'Invisibly disabled and neurodivergent' (an admittedly unwieldy category that will be unpacked more fully in Chapter 2) encompasses a very broad variety of differences, many of them extremely similar to one another in some ways and extremely different from one another in others. Even two students who share the same diagnosis will not always share the same traits, needs, preferences, and experiences. The stigma and anxiety that students may experience around disclosing and discussing their disabilities, furthermore, means that disabled and neurodivergent students are often disconnected from their peers with similar conditions, with no ready means of communicating and comparing experiences. Most invisibly disabled and neurodivergent students know only what it is like to go through college as themselves, and may have little sense of just how common their challenges and observations really are. As a result, they may assume that a particular problem is their own personal failing, rather than a systemic injustice being inflicted upon them by a higher education institution insufficiently equipped to provide them with what they need.

This book, therefore, may also be eye-opening for the same students whose narratives fill it. It is my hope, in fact, that they will learn that others are going through and wishing for the same things that they are, and that they feel increasingly empowered to speak up, join together, and demand change. At the same time, I also hope that this book will serve as a basis of evidence from which higher education faculty, staff, and administrators can not only make adjustments to their own individual practice, but also advocate for more sweeping changes in institution-level committees, task forces, and governance. As the issues and needs identified by the students in these pages are bigger than any one student's story, so they are also larger than any one educator's scope of influence can resolve. Knowing what they are, however, can be our starting point for coalition-building and working together for a better and more equitable environment for all students in the future.

Guiding Principles and Positionality

As an academic librarian educator specializing in instructional technologies and instructional design, my core philosophy in my work sits at the nexus of human-centered design and learner-centered teaching. The two approaches have an interesting set of overlaps and divergences, not always evident to those inexperienced in the ways instructional design brings them into conversation. As described by Norman (2013), among its other proponents, human-centered design emphasizes starting from thorough examination of real people's real needs and habits in order to create objects, spaces, and technologies that will be intuitive for them to use successfully (pp. 8–10). Learner-centered teaching, meanwhile, focuses on changing the instructor's traditional role as leader and authority of the classroom to a supportive role, so that students take primary responsibility for directing and controlling their learning, and their experience and mastery are central (Weimer, 2013). While the contexts, particulars, and goals vary between these two philosophies, a core element is shared between them: both concede most of the power and authority traditionally afforded to the expert (the designer, the educator), and offer renewed recognition and respect for the perspectives of the supposed non-expert (the user, the student), whose success has ostensibly been the point of the exercise all along. To put it bluntly, both are conscious, collaborative exercises in humility, and this fact sometimes causes experts in both fields to balk at their implementation.

To my mind, however, both are imperative if we are actually to develop experiences—learning and otherwise—that meet the needs of those we entered our professions to serve. Toward this end, I chose to begin from the spirit of inquiry that is fundamental to both approaches. Rather than limit my creativity and effectiveness by simply collecting and replicating existing services for invisibly disabled and neurodivergent students, which might or might not actually be best serving the needs of students in practice, I instead sought out available records of students' self-described experiences of higher education, positive and negative. Even as a disabled educator myself, I have only one perspective on what is helpful and harmful in higher education, and I felt that it would be necessary to investigate students' perspectives as thoroughly as possible before I could have any confidence in correctly identifying the problems most in need of solutions.

On a similar note, I have chosen to ground this work in a disability studies in education (DSE) theoretical framework, informed by elements of Disability Critical Race Theory (DisCrit). DSE embraces the social model of disability, and seeks to challenge the prevalent educational understanding of disability as a medicalized deficit to be overcome by the individual. Instead, this understanding positions disability as one of many identities an individual may hold that are systematically marginalized, in intersecting ways, by educational systems and the broader society. Transforming access, equity, and inclusion for disabled people in education is thereby a matter of social justice and liberation, and the disabling impacts that they experience for not conforming to prescriptive expectations of physical and mental functioning are not individual burdens disabled people must bear, but social and systemic failures to meet their needs that must be addressed. DisCrit, meanwhile, marries disability studies and critical race theory perspectives in education research to create a fundamentally intersectional lens, which critically investigates the interactions of race-based and ability-based oppressions in education, particularly with regard to economic and carceral injustice (Connor et al., 2016). These approaches have guided my investigation of students' stories throughout this work, as has my personal commitment to activist principles of disability justice: that the societal structures that oppress disabled people need to be challenged as an inextricable component of challenging all interconnected forms of marginalization, by resisting capitalist commodification and carceral policing of bodies and minds, by rejecting the idea of a 'normal' body and mind and embracing the equal value of all, and by embracing solidarity and collective liberation across identities and communities (Berne, 2015). This radical position shares roots in common with the neurodiversity paradigm, which will be discussed in more detail in the early chapters of this book, and I believe strongly that the level of reform and revolution it advocates will be necessary if we are to pursue true justice and equity for all members of our society.

This book proceeds from the same assumptions, and among them is the principle Berne (2015) outlines of 'Leadership by Those Most Impacted,' a related concept to the one that disability activists have often stated as 'nothing about us without us.' I see myself as undertaking this work in order to lead a conversation as one of those who have been most impacted, but in so doing, I have also let the voices of students lead me. Foregrounding the voices of disabled students, staff, and faculty is a priority that has been identified for the continued course of educational research (Seale, 2017), both in the interest of completeness of information and from a social justice standpoint. It has been one of my primary goals throughout this project, and has greatly informed the research and construction of this book.

Methodological Approach

As alluded to above, the method I selected for the present study was effectively a massive narrative literature review. Given my professional expertise as an academic librarian, which centers on information organization and literature searching and synthesis, combined with the wealth of largely uncompiled qualitative data available, this seemed to be the most suitable way to begin. Rather than conducting my own qualitative research with what would surely be a relatively limited sample size, I could use the existing literature to create a foundation for my and others' future research, by collecting and analyzing the broadest possible variety of rich descriptions of student experiences. With my primary focus on simply capturing student voices where they appeared in the literature, I was less concerned with the quality of research in individual studies than I might otherwise have been, and ultimately chose to broaden my scope to include theses and dissertations, as well as published peer-reviewed books and articles. I also found that the comprehensiveness and specificity of the dissertation format seemed often to lend itself to the types of analysis I was seeking, and this was particularly true of dissertations studying only students with a certain identity or diagnosis.

Because I had a set of specific named conditions or types of conditions in mind for consideration (I discuss the reasoning behind this selection in more detail in Chapter 2), I let those names lead me in the construction of my search terms. My overall search strategy was to conduct seven distinct, overlapping searches, focused on:

1. Generalized terminology such as 'neurodivergent,' 'invisibly disabled,' and similar terms;

2. Dyslexia and variations, including loosely related conditions such as dyscalculia and dyspraxia;

3. Autism and variations, including now-outdated terminology such as 'Asperger's syndrome';

4. Attention deficit hyperactivity disorder or ADHD;

5. A number of variations on the concept of mental illness and mental health disorders, of which I found 'psychiatric disabilities' emerged as the most commonplace;

6. Traumatic brain injuries and variations; and

7. Chronic illness and variations, including names of specific commonly invisible conditions, e.g. Ehlers-Danlos syndrome, inflammatory bowel disease, etc.

In each case, these terms were paired with terms identifying the possible types of study of interest to me, such as interviews, focus groups, qualitative surveys, and similar. I repeated this search across multiple education subject databases, as well as in thesis and dissertation databases, and hand-selected possible candidates from the results. In some cases, I was also able to uncover additional sources from thorough examination of the literature reviews and citations of the studies I included.

Given the sheer amount of literature that could potentially have been encompassed by this approach, I also keenly felt the importance of limiting the scope of my review only to what was of primary interest. For the process of selecting studies from my initial results sets, I developed a set of stringent criteria for inclusion, as follows:

- Only studies that presented student voices directly were added. These could take the form of summaries of and quotations from interviews, survey responses, or similar, but quantitative survey responses were not included.

- Studies were excluded if their findings related only to coursework, teaching faculty, university-level accommodations, or combinations of these. While these studies would be useful for teaching faculty or for disability services staff, they would have little relevance for others in academic support roles with minimal influence over these factors, including myself. Many findings of this study do relate to coursework and accommodations, but these are generally recorded in the context of more broadly applicable findings and conclusions.

- Studies were also excluded if their primary focus was the transition from high school to college, mainly because this is a broad enough topic in itself to warrant a separate investigation. As with coursework and accommodations, some information is included here on challenges for new college students, but the primary focus is on students who are established at the postsecondary level.

- Studies were also excluded if their primary focus was on evaluating the success of a particular program or intervention, since my goal was to focus on broader experiences rather than students' reactions to specific attempts at solutions.

- Studies were considered from all types of postsecondary institution and from any geographic location. As I was only able to consider English-language studies, the majority of included studies were conducted with students from the United States, Canada, the United Kingdom, and Australia, although some studies from mainland European nations, African nations, and a few others were also included.

- In general, only studies published in 2011 or later were considered, as inclusive practices change and develop rapidly and therefore it was preferable to only examine contributions from the preceding decade. This cutoff date was flexible, however, with some slightly earlier studies included if they were found to be sufficiently cited by and significant to subsequent research.

These guidelines served to define the main body of literature used in this study, for a total of approximately 180 articles, book chapters, and dissertations. I worked systematically through the results of each individual search, examining findings and identifying recurring themes, both for students in each grouping and held in common across multiple groupings. My findings have been organized by theme into the chapters that make up Part II of this book.

It should be noted explicitly, however, that as much of a wealth of information as I was able to synthesize using this approach, it is severely limited in at least one respect: the predominance of white study participants. A substantive critique of the existing literature on disability in higher education is its centering the experiences of white students while failing to meaningfully engage with the impacts of race on disabled students (Stapleton & James, 2020), and I have found this to affect the vast majority of studies I examined, with many describing overwhelmingly or entirely white participant pools, if the race of participants is identified at all. I eagerly anticipate future growth in the body of literature on the experiences of disabled students of color, as this is a significant gap in dire need of being addressed. Working with the available literature in the meantime, however, while I doubt I could fully compensate for this concern, I have made a deliberate effort to address it. A full chapter has been devoted to literature that would otherwise have been out of scope for this review, but that reveals intersectional considerations that may impact disabled and neurodivergent students with other marginalized identities. I have also taken care to note ways in which minoritized racial identities may specifically impact student experiences reported in the literature, wherever they arise. Even so, the whiteness of the participants in the core literature under discussion here should remain front of mind when considering its conclusions, and the relative absence of the voices of students of color necessarily limits any claims I can make as to their generalizability.

Structure

Part I, Foundations, begins by establishing the context into which this work enters, as well as its terms and parameters. Chapter 1 discusses the landscape of higher education as it pertains to disabled students in general, and invisibly disabled and neurodivergent students in particular. It provides a brief overview of the history of disabled students' inclusion in higher education, including relevant movements and legislation, and then addresses the major thematic barriers that disabled students still encounter to this day: the power structures inherent in higher education in its present form, the restraints on the capacity of institutions and their staff, neoliberal attitudes and academic capitalism in colleges and universities, and specific stigmas around learning and psychiatric disabilities in college students. With these factors in mind, Chapter 2 outlines the terminology and categories in use to name and organize neurodivergent and invisibly disabled students in this work, and the reasoning behind their selection. It also addresses the limitations of these rhetorical constructions, and the nuances that make them less simple in practical fact than they may appear on the page.

In Part II, Challenges, the main body of research is laid out in a series of themed chapters. Chapter 3 discusses students' experiences of institutional systems and disability services offices and personnel, including the overall challenges presented by institutions and their accommodations processes, and issues around choices of learning modality, as well as the tensions of self-advocacy, disclosure, and help-seeking that students experience, such as the barriers and benefits around acknowledging their conditions and seeking support, issues around diagnosis, and the role of disability identity. Chapter 4 describes students' experiences in the curriculum and classroom, and what serves them most and least in terms of faculty attitudes, the intrinsic academic strengths and weaknesses associated with the categories discussed here, and different elements of course structure and instructional delivery. Chapter 5 discusses student life experiences outside of the curriculum, meanwhile, including social issues and relationships with peers, mental health challenges, and the physical environment on campus. Chapter 6 then turns particular attention to intersectional considerations, including how disabled and neurodivergent students' experiences are impacted by additionally minoritized racial and ethnic, gender, and LGBTQ+ identities, as well as by trauma experiences, which are relatively common for disabled and neurodivergent students and even more so if they are multiply marginalized.

Part III, Directions for Positive Change, finally shifts the focus from narratives of student experiences to distill some of the most critical needs for support that those narratives have identified, and examples of promising practices from the literature that have been or could be implemented to address those needs. Chapter 7 addresses strategies in this area for addressing student needs within the curriculum, including considerations around time flexibility, removing barriers to accommodations, assistive technologies, proactive outreach and intervention strategies, and mentoring and coaching programs. Chapter 8 looks instead at strategies for needs outside the curriculum, which include financial and career support, improving the campus social climate, facilitating student connections to social support networks, mental and physical health care, and skill-building and information support. Finally, the Conclusions revisit the larger core concerns that must be addressed in light of all of this information, including the urgency of improving higher education, given its benefits, and the need to trust students as our partners in this work, and to identify necessary directions for future action and research in this area.

As a final logistical note, this book primarily employs parenthetical citations in the text, in accordance with U.S. conventions of educational research and for speed and ease of referencing. Due to its nature as a broad literature review, however, there are areas where a large number of references are included to support a single point. Therefore, parenthetical citations are used when citing three or fewer references, but in cases where more than three references are included in a single citation, for readability these have been removed to footnotes.

PART I

FOUNDATIONS

1. The Higher Education Landscape

Higher education and academic settings are particularly fraught with complexities for students with all types of disabilities. The history of disabled students' participation in higher education is shorter than many-able bodied people would expect, and it has required great effort to bring it to the point where it currently stands. Neither, for that matter, can it be claimed that higher education is a welcoming and supportive environment for students with disabilities at the present moment, much less that they have the same opportunities to succeed in colleges and universities as other students do. It is critical to begin this discussion by acknowledging first that, through the great efforts of many activists, success in higher education is more achievable for students with disabilities than it has been in the past, and second that it is still not as achievable as it needs to be. Those of us who work in higher education must be willing to recognize that we still have much to learn and much work to do before we can serve students with disabilities equitably in our institutions, and that begins with looking candidly at where the problems have been and still are in the higher education landscape.

Disability in Higher Education History

In the introduction to *Academic Ableism: Disability and Higher Education*, Dolmage (2017) argues that higher education has in many ways defined itself in opposition to disability: that 'higher education' presents itself as an elite place to demonstrate ability, both mental and physical, while the institutions of confinement, labor, and remediation that were seen as appropriate for disabled people in past centuries were understood to represent a kind of opposing 'lower education' (p. 3). Elsewhere in

    https://doi.org/10.11647/OBP.0420.01

the same work, Dolmage also connects higher education's exclusion of disabled people with another disturbing aspect of academic history in the U.S.: the embrace and propagation of eugenics by North American scholars, particularly in the first decades of the twentieth century (pp. 11–20, 49–53). The pseudoscience of supposedly pursuing human perfection by eliminating 'undesirable' traits and promoting 'positive' ones (inevitably associated with whiteness, maleness, heterosexuality, ability, and other privileged and dominant identities, while 'undesirable' encompassed all alternatives) played a significant part in establishing the modes of study, norms, and principles of much of the modern academy:

> Not only did eugenics actually reshape the North American population through things like immigration restriction, not only did it reshape families through its campaigns for 'better breeding,' not only did it reshape bodies through medical intervention, but it reshaped how North Americans thought about bodies and minds.

> Academia is implicated very deeply in this history. Academia was the place from which eugenic 'science' gained its funding and legitimization so that eugenicists could undertake massive projects in both 'positive' and 'negative' eugenics. But the university was also itself a laboratory for 'positive' eugenics, a place where the 'right' combinations of genes could be brought together ('the better families') and where eugenic ideals and values could be conveyed to the future teachers, lawyers, doctors, and other professionals on campus. (Dolmage, 2018, p. 13)

As Dolmage also describes, many university buildings to this day stand literally on the bones of those who were subject to inhumane experimentation and other abuses toward eugenicist ends (pp. 49–50). Academia as the laboratory of eugenics resulted in numerous real and horrifyingly violent consequences for people with disabilities, alongside members of other marginalized communities. Indeed, eugenicist ideas of disabled people's deficiencies were also used to implicate minoritized racial and ethnic identities, by claiming these groups to be inherently associated with physical and mental impairments in order to support dispossession and discrimination (pp. 14–16). This was true of North American people of color, particularly African Americans and indigenous communities, and of immigrants of color, as Dolmage (2018) also discusses in more detail in *Disabled Upon Arrival: Eugenics, Immigration, and the Construction of Race and Disability*. Well into the twentieth century, claims like these were a part of accepted scholarly discourse, while disability was seen as fundamentally incompatible with the academy, and disabled students as having no place in postsecondary education. In the United States, in particular, this dreadful legacy of higher education has yet to be truly confronted, as evidenced by how seldom discussed and little known it remains to this day.

It was only through a great deal of courageous work and activism that this perceived incompatibility began to shift, and that the possibility of the disabled college student—let alone the disabled scholar—began to be constructed. Although there were other catalysts as well, four main factors may have contributed most to this transition in the United States context:

1. Advocacy for d/Deaf education;

2. College attendance by disabled veterans prompted by the G.I. Bill;

3. The Independent Living Movement; and

4. Several key pieces of U.S. legislation regarding the rights of disabled people.

d/Deaf Education and Higher Education

In the United States, Deaf communities have represented one of the oldest forces advocating for rights for a disabled community, even if that advocacy has been complicated and troubled in a number of ways. A relatively cohesive and independent Deaf culture has existed since at least the 19th century, and specifically d/Deaf educational institutions have played a major role in helping this community-building to occur—a role that has resulted in serious and detrimental pushback against these same institutions.

The long-time bastion of d/Deaf higher education in the United States is Gallaudet University, previously Gallaudet College and the National Deaf-Mute College. The institution was established in 1817 as the American Asylum for the Education and Instruction of Deaf and Dumb Persons, co-founded by hearing American minister Thomas Hopkins Gallaudet and Deaf French teacher Laurent Clerc, to disseminate French progressive methods in d/Deaf education in North America (Edwards, 2001, pp. 60–61). Clerc was profoundly deaf and communicated entirely through sign, which was also the preferred style of education in the French institutions in which he had been taught, and as a result the American Asylum also followed these methods. Teachers were expected to be fluent in Deaf community-originating naturalistic sign patterns as well as more formal sign language, which Edwards (2001) points out was not only quite revolutionary at the time, but has been for much of subsequent history (pp. 61–62). Deaf education flourished under this approach, and Gallaudet went on to be president of the Columbia Institution for the Deaf, Dumb, and Blind, which in 1864 was authorized to award the first college degrees to d/Deaf students (Fleischer & Zames, 2011, p. 17).

By the turn of the 20th century, however, these successes had met with a backlash. As Edwards (2001) suggests, Deaf people's possession of the shared language of sign, which education in sign helped to propagate, enabled the development of collective Deaf identity and independent community—which was discomforting and concerning to educational activists of the day, who were steeped in ableist views of any disability as an inherently dehumanizing deficit, and not a suitable basis for community and pride (pp. 74–75). The source of critics' dismay seems to have been entirely that Deaf people embraced one another and Deafness, rather than rejecting their difference with shame and striving to be as much like hearing people as possible (Edwards, 2001, p. 74). The destructive consequence of this reaction was the promotion and eventual adoption of what was known as the oralist method of deaf education (as opposed to the manualist method of using hand signs). Rather than allowing deaf education to be led by and conducted in Deaf people's own language, oralism insisted that d/Deaf students should be taught to learn and behave as much as possible as though they were hearing, and that attaining spoken language should be their primary goal. This approach focused singularly on integrating d/Deaf people into hearing society, which, as Edwards (2001) suggests, was intended to also serve the goal of defusing the perceived threat of Deaf community-building. Not only was this seen as a rhetorical threat to able-bodied supremacy, but as a physical threat to the eugenicist elimination of the perceived deficit of deafness: Deaf people in community would be more likely to marry and procreate with one another, which it was feared would produce more Deaf people (Fleischer & Zames, 2011, p. 17). Furthermore, as Fleischer and Zames (2011) also note, oralism simply was not a cognitively appropriate learning method for d/Deaf children, as it involved insisting that they communicate from a young age only in ways that were uncomfortable and unnatural for all and impossible for many; once proponents were able to successfully achieve their widespread adoption, oralist methods significantly impaired generations of d/Deaf students' language acquisition, cognitive development, and educational efficacy (pp. 15–16). Not only did this shift in d/Deaf education strive to break up Deaf community, it was also to the detriment of d/Deaf education and therefore also to their social participation and economic success, making it a form of systemic oppression that persisted into the latter half of the 20th century.

As a number of authors have pointed out, however, neither should the relative cohesion and strength of historical Deaf communities be misconstrued as lost utopian perfection. Deaf communities in particular have been prone to divisions and internal oppressions, in part as a defensively conservative response to oppression from without. Racial segregation and discrimination, particularly anti-Blackness, have been as much a part of the history of d/Deaf education in the United States as that of hearing education, and the greatest successes of d/Deaf education in the 19th century were in reality largely the successes of *white* d/Deaf education. African American students were instead consistently relegated to inferior resources and facilities, and so segregated from white Deaf students that their sign dialects developed significantly differently, to the point that they lacked the advantage of a shared language (Burch & Sutherland, 2006, p. 141; Nielsen, 2012, pp. 136–137). Extremely conservative gender roles also developed in Deaf communities, often as a defense of Deaf men's remaining social power in response to hearing and oralist oppression, which severely limited Deaf women's participation in Deaf culture and in society in general (Burch, 2001; Burch & Sutherland, 2006). As beneficial as Gallaudet University and higher education were to parts of Deaf society, those with access to them tended to be elite members of the community, entrenching classist divisions in the community as well and keeping the greatest benefits from working-class d/Deaf people (Burch & Sutherland, 2006). It is worth noting, also, that the pressure to integrate with hearing society and reject disability identity exemplified by the oralist movement also appears to have taken a lasting toll, in the form of Deaf communities' historical resistance to early coalition-building with other disabled

activists. For example, Nielsen (2012) points to Deaf leaders' refusal
to ally with disabled activist organizations against employment
discrimination in the 1930s, out of willingness to accept discrimination
in employment against disabled people as long as Deaf people were not
considered 'disabled people,' as well as fear of marginalization within a
broader community by hearing disabled people (p. 136).

Over time, though, Deaf communities' embrace of disability identity
and pride has increased, and some of these attitudinal shifts have also
been associated with Deaf education in general, and Gallaudet University
in particular. For example, Nielsen (2012) also points to the 1988 student
protest campaign at Gallaudet—which, as Shapiro (2004) notes, should
also be recognized as definitively an *alumni* protest campaign (pp.
75–76)—titled the Deaf President Now (DPN) campaign. This protest
led to the institution of the first Deaf president of the university, and was
one example of the movement toward positive disability pride in the U.S.
in the 1980s. As problematic as some of the stratification with regard to
d/Deaf education has been, the fact that such a noteworthy campaign
for representation in leadership was centered around a higher education
institution should point to how important a role postsecondary learning
has played in the life of Deaf communities.

Disabled Veterans and Higher Education

The U.S. Soldier Rehabilitation Act of 1918 and Vocational Rehabilitation
Act of 1920, passed after the end of World War I, attempted to secure
some educational support and services for disabled veterans of the war,
although the focus was almost exclusively on job preparation (Bryan,
2010, p. 217). The capacity of the programs created was also poorly
matched to demand, and the impact was mixed as a result (Madaus
et al., 2009; Madaus, 2011). The legislation that had a much more
substantial and lasting impact on American higher education, however,
was the G.I. Bill of Rights, or the Serviceman's Readjustment Act of
1944, which financially supported honorably discharged servicepeople
in pursuing higher education. As in the wake of World War II, many
of those meeting this description had been disabled in combat to some
degree; this led to an unprecedented influx of disabled students into
U.S. colleges and universities—for which the vast majority of these
institutions were neither equipped nor enthused (Pelka, 2011, p. 94).

Programs began to be developed at a number of institutions, including the University of California at Los Angeles, the University of Illinois, the City College of New York, the University of Minnesota, and others, most often in conjunction with nearby veterans' hospitals or associations (Madaus et al., 2009; Madaus, 2011). The majority of these programs, however, were still significantly lacking by 1950, when the American Council on Education (ACE) commissioned a report on veterans with disabilities attending postsecondary institutions, which concluded that 'colleges and universities were not prepared to meet the needs of veterans with disabilities, and pointed to examples from veterans who did not receive services, even at institutions that stated that such services were provided' (Madaus et al., 2009). To read these paraphrased words from as early as 1950 should be sobering, as they identify a theme that has been common throughout the history of all students with disabilities in higher education, up to and including the present day.

One of the most successful and widely recognized programs of the day was that of the University of Illinois, and even this example, as a case study, illustrates many of the problems that were inherent in these early approaches. The University of Illinois program, under the directorship of Timothy Nugent, began at an ad hoc campus in Galesburg, Illinois, which was converted from a newly-built hospital that was found not to be needed after the end of the war (Pelka, 2011, p. 95). The program faced skepticism, discrimination, and hostility from the university and from the surrounding community, and within a few years the university sought to close down the entire Galesburg campus, citing budgetary reasons. With support from multiple veterans' organizations, the students and program leaders demonstrated in the state capital and on the main campus in Champaign, and eventually university administration allowed the program to move to the main campus as an 'experiment,' which was underfunded and poorly supported (Pelka, 2011, pp. 96–97). As part of his programs for wheelchair-using students, Nugent instituted wheelchair athletics and training in independent living activities, and procured a set of lift-equipped buses for student transportation, despite so much resistance from administrators that leveraging organizations of students' families to put pressure on the university was often the only path to success (Pelka, 2011). Both Nugent and later students in the program also worked to improve the accessibility of buildings on campus and in the surrounding town. The program provided tremendous opportunities for many students who would have few other options at the time.

Even so, multiple former students in Pelka (2011) describe their experiences with Nugent's program in complicated terms, recounting its value to them but also how much its director insisted that students in the program participate entirely unsupported, without aid from medical assistants, help from others on campus, or even the use of power wheelchairs (pp. 105, 109, 111–112). Nugent's corresponding narratives express obvious pride in these same insistences, suggesting that they fostered independence in students, and it is true to a degree that his high expectations of disabled people and recognition of their capacity for independence would have been remarkable among common attitudes at the time. Still, as activist Mary Lou Breslin—who experienced Nugent's tenure—puts it, this does not account for 'the whole concept of the level playing field, of how attendants made people physically independent [...]. Only people who were physically able to play basketball, do wheelchair tricks, or be a cheerleader were accepted' (Pelka, 2011, p. 109). While the program's strictures may have provided those who were able to meet them with pride in their accomplishment, they also left behind far more of those no less capable but simply with different physical needs.

Pelka (2011) describes Nugent's requirements of students as 'a bridge between the paternalism of the vocational rehabilitation movement of the 1940s and '50s and the modern era of disability rights' (p. 95): his work helped to prepare some leaders for a future of greater liberation, but was in many ways steeped in past destructive attitudes about disability. His approach is emblematic of what is called the 'whole man' rehabilitation philosophy to which Pelka alludes, based on the work of Dr. Henry Kessler and Dr. Howard Rusk with wounded servicepeople after World Wars I and II, focusing on rehabilitation and independence in every area of life rather than treating the injury alone (Fleischer & Zames, 2011, p. 172). While this movement was in many ways positive for modern understandings of rehabilitation and disability, its primary focus was on independence achieved by the actions of the disabled person, rather than changes to increase accessibility in social services and institutions, which set a burdensome precedent for the ways that disability is addressed even to this day. It is also worth noting that, while in cases like the University of Illinois the need to support disabled veterans led to program advancements that could also serve disabled civilians like Breslin, communities of disabled veterans were also much more invested in their identity as veterans than in solidarity with other disabled people. Veterans' organizations went so far as lobbying for separate and special laws stipulating different supports and treatments for disabled veterans and disabled civilians, rejecting (as with Deaf communities) any coalition-building with other seekers for disability justice (Fleischer & Zames, 2011, p. 171). While it is important to acknowledge that the need to support disabled veterans opened the door for other disabled students, it is also important to note that the door was certainly not opened all the way for all students equally, and also that some who had entered were invested in pushing it shut again behind them.

Furthermore, while programs and services continued to develop for veterans after the Korean and Vietnam Wars, many campuses continued to be completely inaccessible and not to accept disabled students at all. Support for veteran benefits was also significantly cut by the Reagan administration in the 1980s, substantially impacting the access to services that were available by the end of the Persian Gulf War (Madaus et al., 2009).

The Independent Living Movement and Higher Education

In addition to being a severe restriction of disabled people's rights in itself, one of the greatest barriers to disabled organizing and activism prior to the mid-twentieth century was the common confinement of people with disabilities in medical institutions. In the 1950s and 1960s in the U.S., however, medical procedures and technology began to reach a point where people with many kinds of disabilities were able to have more physical mobility, and more avenues opened to other types of independence (Scotch, 1988, p. 164). These decades saw a few test cases of what Fleischer and Zames (2011) refer to as 'deinstitutionalization,' where people with severe mobility impairments began to receive support first to create more positive spaces for themselves within medical institutions, and then to move out of them altogether and into the mainstream of society (pp. 33–34). These efforts proceeded alongside increasing pushes for legislation to support disabled people in pursuing education, work, and independence as well, such as the Rehabilitation Act of 1973.

One significant result of this direction, in the 1970s, was the establishment of independent living centers: communities for disabled people to reside in, with resources and services available to reduce barriers, where the emphasis was placed on empowering disabled people toward autonomy and personal fulfillment (Winter, 2003). The history of these centers is also closely tied to higher education, since the first Center for Independent Living (CIL) was established in 1972 as an outgrowth of student activism at the University of California at Berkeley. The CIL was founded and run by disabled Berkeley students and graduates, led by Ed Roberts, a polio survivor with severe respiratory and mobility impairments, and also a dedicated student activist. Roberts fought a legal battle to be allowed to attend Berkeley with the use of a wheelchair and portable respirator, and his success attracted the attention and eventual attendance of more students with significant disabilities (Fleischer & Zames, 2011; Pelka, 2011). Appropriate housing for Roberts, able to accommodate his needs and his eight-hundred-pound iron lung, was not available on the university campus proper, so Roberts and the others with similar needs who came to attend the university were housed in a ward of Cowell Hospital, at the edge of campus (Fleischer & Zames, 2011, p. 38). Roberts also quickly became deeply involved in social justice activism at the university, a context that surely helped him to see his own struggle and those of his peers as a civil rights issue and a case of societal discrimination, rather than an interior deficit to be overcome (Pelka, 2011, p. 197). The community they formed at Cowell Hospital served as the base of a group calling itself the 'Rolling Quads,' which continued to push for greater access at the university and beyond, leading to the 1970 opening of the government-funded Physically Disabled Students' Program (PDSP) at Berkeley (Pelka, 2011). This program became a source of support services and resources for disabled people in the surrounding community as well as students, hiring disabled counselors and providing a wide range of services up to and including wheelchair repair (Shapiro, 1994, p. 51). When it was clear that there was a need for a similar support structure for alumni and community members, Roberts and other PDSP students founded the CIL to meet it (Pelka, 2011, pp. 197–198). The CIL offered disabled people a wide variety of services and supports, many through peer support networks and community, and it became the center of some of the boldest disability social justice activism throughout the 1970s (Fleischer & Zames, 2011; Pelka, 2011). This was especially true when political backlash, citing the costs of supporting people with disabilities, threatened many of the gains the PDSP, CIL, and other organizations had made (Shapiro, 1994, pp. 70–73). In time, other independent living centers were also established across the country, leading not only to practical benefits for those with access to them, but an increased sense of empowerment and pride as well (Winters, 2003).

While the CIL and a number of other independent living centers that arose may have done so initially within universities, in large part their inception was more in spite of higher education administration than because of it—as could be said of much of the student activism of the 1960s and 1970s. Roberts had to overcome UC Berkeley's resistance to admitting him in the first place for other students to realize they could achieve the same, and it was the students themselves who had the perseverance to attend in spite of the difficulties, and the courage and advocacy skills to make changes. It certainly was not the university, which offered them so few resources in the process that they had to reside in a hospital ward instead of a dormitory. This has remained an unfortunately persistent reality within higher education: institutions tend to balk at changing discriminatory systems and policies until pressured, sometimes aggressively, by especially strong advocates.

The case of the CIL is particularly impressive because of how much was accomplished, and, as Bryan (2006) notes, because of how much of it was led by students with particularly severe physical limitations and restrictions (pp. 43–44). It is important to note, however, that the story of the Berkeley CIL—and of others like it—is not a simple tale of individualistic triumph. For one thing, much of what enabled the development of the PDSP and the CIL, and similar independent living centers, was in fact government funding, largely through 1978 subsidies to the Rehabilitation Act of 1973 (Bryan, 2006, p. 45; Fleischer & Zames, 2011, p. 46). Support at the level of national social services was critical to the establishment of independent living centers. It was also, unfortunately, insufficient to provide universal access to independent living centers, or to other resources for disabled people.

As Nielsen (2012) notes, in a large number of cases the movement to deinstitutionalization has, instead, effectively been a movement to the abandonment of people with disabilities due to lack of support, lack of services, and becoming unhoused, particularly in cases of psychiatric disabilities (p. 164). Historically, independent living centers have also not served all people with disabilities equally. African American activist Donald Galloway, for example, has recounted Roberts' and the CIL's centering of people with physical and mobility disabilities over those with other types of disability (Pelka, 2011, p. 220). More importantly, he also notes the lack of diversity in the CIL's leadership, and that they were reluctant to boost marginalized voices within the community, or attend to the intersections of where multiply marginalized community members, such as Black disabled people, are disproportionately impacted by disability (Pelka, 2011, pp. 220–221).

Legislation: The Education of All Handicapped Children Act, Section 504, and the Americans with Disabilities Act

At the same time that disabled veterans were claiming access to higher education, meanwhile, parents of children with disabilities were organizing into advocacy groups for their children's right to education. Later referred to as the 'parents' movement,' this work began in the 1930s, and only burgeoned through the 1940s and 1950s with support from disabled veterans seeking additional services for their families; it was also eventually emboldened by *Brown v. Board of Education* and other efforts toward racial civil rights in education (Pelka, 2011, p. 131). Throughout the 1960s, parent and family activists fought legal battles against continuing discrimination toward disabled people, in education but also in other critical areas, including abuse in care institutions for children with cognitive disabilities, cerebral palsy, and similar conditions. The successes and networks built by these efforts eventually supported direct lobbying in Washington, D.C., providing grassroots backing to enable the passage of major legislation (Pelka, 2011, p. 141). The most significant accomplishment at this point in the movement's life was the 1975 passage of the Education of All Handicapped Children Act, reestablished in 1990 as the Individuals with Disabilities Education Act, or IDEA (Fleischer & Zames, 2011, p. 184).

The core of IDEA is the requirement that all eligible children and young people, including those with disabilities, must have access to 'a free, appropriate public education,' which includes special education and services meeting state standards, directed by an individualized education plan (IEP) developed by experts and parents, and provided publicly with no additional charge to families of disabled children (Bryan, 2006, p. 61). Another critical component of IDEA has been the concept of the 'least restrictive environment,' by which the act proposed to end the separation and isolation of disabled students, and integrate them into educational environments with their nondisabled peers (Pelka, 2011, p. 144). Helpfully, activists were able to argue for this measure by comparing the issue to that of racial school segregation (Fleischer & Zames, 2011, p. 185). This significant legislative achievement had major implications for primary and secondary education in the U.S., although as Fleischer and Zames (2011) describe, enforcement would prove to be a more complicated matter.

In its initial form, IDEA was focused on primary and secondary education, and had far fewer implications for the postsecondary level. This changed, however, with additional legislation only a few years later. In 1977, also thanks to the grassroots organizing of disabled activists, Section 504 of the Vocational Rehabilitation Act was signed into law. This section protects disabled people nationally from disability-based discrimination in organizations receiving federal funding—although the logistics of enforcement in private industry proved more elusive than in federal agencies (Bryan, 2010, p. 234). Furthermore, Section E specifically requires both public and private higher education institutions to consider qualified applicants regardless of ability status, and to provide necessary accommodations and support for students with disabilities (Madaus, 2011, p. 9). In close succession, Section 504 was followed in 1978 by amendments to IDEA, then the Education of All Handicapped Children Act, part of which addressed higher education for disabled students, in the context of requiring schools to aid them in the transition to adulthood (Madaus, 2011, p. 9). Together, these two additions to the existing legislation made a significant stride toward guaranteeing access to higher education for disabled students.

Unfortunately, in the years afterward, enforcement of Section 504 proved elusive, including in higher education. Only after more protesting, direct action, and pressure on government officials—including a sit-in demonstration in Washington, D.C. supported by LGBT and Chicano activists, as well as the Black Panthers—were enforcement regulations enacted, threatening the funding of organizations found to discriminate on the basis of disability (Nielsen, 2012, pp. 168–169). Postsecondary institutions responded to the requirements of Section 504 in particular with initial trepidation and hostility, fearing, as Madaus (2011) puts it, 'closure because of costs related to compliance' (p. 9). Even so, the requirements were now law, and as Scott (1988) points out, their construction of disability as a legally protected category and a basis of discrimination, like race, also had possibly equally significant effects on disability rights and organizing moving forward (p. 167). Scott also notes that another highly significant element of these definitions of disability enshrined in law is that, rather than having been set by government officials and medical experts as in past instances, these were crafted and in some cases written by advocates from the disability rights movement itself (p. 168). From multiple perspectives, these legislative achievements were vindications of the principle of 'nothing about us without us' that has been a key component of disability activism.

As much as Section 504 and the amendments to IDEA helped push forward disability rights in higher education, the 1990 Americans with Disabilities Act (ADA), along with its other expansions of disability rights, also played a significant role in increasing what was possible for disabled postsecondary students (Madaus, 2011, p. 10). The road to ADA's passage was a long, complex, and arduous one, requiring tremendous contributions from all of those who advocated for it, and has been documented in a number of disability rights histories already. In short, disability rights advocates had built significant political skills and coalitions with other civil rights movements around the passage of Section 504, which set them up for success in further endeavors (Bryan, 2006, pp. 64–66). Seasoned disability rights advocates built relationships in Washington that allowed them to participate in the drafting, supporting, and lobbying that were necessary for the bill to be passed. As Davis (2015) alludes to, much of ADA's success seems to have come from clever use of the unique nature of disability as an identity: it can belong to anyone, anywhere, at any time, and therefore even among Washington elites, unexpected allies tended to pop up in unexpected places (p. 8). Much of Pelka's (2011) lengthy recounting of ADA process follows the same pattern, again and again: disability rights advocates secured support from one political insider after another, each with some personal connection to disability. Advocates leveraged this advantage carefully to pass—with surprisingly bipartisan support—a relatively powerful piece of legislation acknowledging the history of discrimination against disability, and establishing broad protections against it in the future.

Of the five titles of ADA, Title II, 'Public Services,' pertains most directly to public higher education, and Title III, 'Public Accommodations and Services Operated by Private Entities' to private higher education. The responsibilities indicated by these sections led to further growth in accommodations, services, and programs for disabled students from 1990 onward. Disability services increasingly emerged as a professional area within higher education, leading to the establishment of the professional organization Association on Higher Education and Disability; professionals in this area placed increasing value on students' self-determination and the principles of Universal Design, which were borrowed from their origins in architecture (Madaus, 2011, p. 10).

By no means have all of the developments since ADA was passed represented forward progress, however. As Winter (2003) notes, as with Section 504, compliance with ADA has often been lacking and enforcement has proven a perpetual challenge, and many of the terms and definitions in ADA (e.g. 'reasonable accommodation') have been subject to considerable dispute, confusion, and interpretation. Furthermore, Madaus (2011) acknowledges that there has been a significant legal backlash to ADA's push for services for disabled students since the late 1990s and early 2000s, including a number of court cases whose outcomes have generally favored more restrictive, conservative interpretations of ADA's requirements (p. 11). As Madaus's writing demonstrates, in 2011 significant concerns and issues persisted in the field of serving students with disabilities, most of which are still quite familiar to higher education professionals over a decade later, such as:

- Continuing legislative adjustments, such as the 2009 Americans with Disabilities Act Amendments Act (ADAAA);

- New entering populations particularly of neurodivergent students, those with learning disabilities, and those with psychiatric conditions;

- Continued developments in serving disabled veteran students; and

- Changes in available assistive technology (Madaus, 2011, pp. 11–13).

Neither are these the only issues still facing neurodivergent and disabled students in higher education.

Persistent Barriers for Disabled Students in Higher Education

There are a number of factors in higher education, perhaps even intrinsic to higher education in its current form, which work against access and equity for students with disabilities. While these likely extend well beyond the factors described below, these are some of the most relevant specifically for students who are neurodivergent and invisibly disabled, in the particular ways to be discussed in this book.

Power Structures

The systems and structures of higher education are, in many ways, built to reinforce power imbalances and inequalities that exist more broadly in society at large, privileging the already privileged and marginalizing the already marginalized. For one thing, many of the ways in which colleges and universities function have remained much the same, sometimes uninterrogated, since past centuries, in which further education was explicitly intended only for elite, wealthy, white men. While this expectation may (usually) no longer be overt, it has left an imprint on the assumptions and requirements of higher education that has proven difficult to eradicate, and that now clashes bitterly with the current function of a college degree as a near-universal requirement for professional and economic success. The standard workload and deadline expectations of the average college class, for example, assume that students can, and should, make coursework the central priority of their lives, rather than facing working-class realities of juggling multiple responsibilities for survival. The typical reading and writing requirements for many disciplines assume that students have been raised and educated in environments of white academic English, with neurotypical levels of facility in processing, understanding, and reproducing language. The need to petition for financial and academic support as a special accommodation assumes that the norm is a student who is primarily supported by family, rather than needing to be a primary support for family. The typical classroom assumes that the 'normal student' can walk between narrow and sometimes stepped rows of seats, see distant chalkboards and projector screens, hear and instantly understand lecturing faculty, sit still, concentrate, avoid drowsiness, take notes on the fly, and tolerate prolonged social exposure, among other expectations. These assumptions are not made maliciously, and sometimes there are good reasons for them to be made. They are still, however, assumptions of characteristics that are not universal, and inequitably advantage some students, who have always had relative advantages, over others, who have always been at a relative disadvantage. Nor is this the only way that the typical business of higher education reinforces existing inequities, particularly in the present moment.

In *Academic Ableism,* Dolmage (2017) repeatedly refers to the metaphor of 'steep steps': the tendency for higher education institutions to place material, imposing architectural structures at key points of entry and access on campus, which also serve as metaphorical ascents that supposedly only the most capable can climb. These structures then also bar access to academia and the advancement it should offer, both physically and metaphorically, to those who don't fit its expectations— including the expectation of being able-bodied: 'The university pulls some people slowly up the stairs, and it arranges others at the bottom of this steep incline. The university also steps our society, reinforcing hierarchies and divisions' (p. 45). This claim builds on previous work, such as Charlton's (1998) foundational *Nothing About Us Without Us: Disability Oppression and Empowerment*, which describes the ways that (mainly primary and secondary) educational systems reproduce and reinscribe systems of power from the broader society. This includes funnelling students with disabilities into different and implicitly lesser pedagogical and professional paths:

> Special Education, like so many other reforms won by the popular
> struggle, has been transformed from a way to increase the probability
> that students with disabilities will get some kind of an education into a
> badge of inferiority and a rule-bound, bureaucratic process of separating
> and then warehousing millions of young people that the dominant
> culture has no need for. While this process is uneven, with a minority
> benefiting from true inclusionary practices, the overarching influences of
> race and class preclude any significant and meaningful equalization of
> educational opportunities. (p. 33)

Nor, as Charlton and others would argue, is this out of line with how
education proceeds in general. Propping up systems of social power
and privilege is part of the core function of education, including
higher education, in the way it currently exists and as a legacy of its
historical roots. Giroux (2011) identifies the influence on academia of
what he calls the 'culture of positivism': the ideological tendency, held
over particularly from 19th- and 20th-century scientific approaches to
scholarship, to value only 'objective' truth and knowledge, and ignore
the ways that even what seem to be 'objective' conclusions are colored
by human perception, bias, and error. Adhering to this ideology makes
it possible to claim that education even in history and social phenomena
can, and should, proceed in the absence of context, nuance, politics, and
social values, which in turn helps to reinforce existing power structures
and exert social control over the educated even while obscuring the
fact that it is doing so (pp. 36–39). Existing systems of power and
marginalization are thus treated as self-evident matters of common
sense, and go unchallenged.

One of the starkest examples and results of how power structures
are reproduced in education is the prevalence of carceral attitudes in
schools. Discipline, punishment, and policing have become increasingly
and disturbingly standard elements of U.S. primary and secondary
education over recent decades, and to the detriment of students'
educational outcomes and actual safety, particularly for students who are
already marginalized. In their introduction to a special issue of *American
Behavioral Scientist* on carcerality and educational access, Huerta and
Britton (2022) describe the negative impacts that contact with carceral
systems in primary and secondary schooling have on students' later
college success, and how overuse of discipline and policing in schools
increases these impacts, disproportionately along lines of gender and

race (p. 1312). In a later article in the same issue, Dizon et al. (2022) identify how carceral systems and structures are used to control and surveil students who are perceived as threats to the interests of the institution, economic and otherwise—which, in practice, are perceptions that are disproportionately likely to fall on Black students. Neither do explicit policing and criminalization need to be present in classrooms for educational institutions to perpetuate carceral attitudes, as Moro (2020) incisively articulates in his more colorfully titled blog post 'Against Cop Shit.' What he defines as 'any pedagogical technique or technology that presumes an adversarial relationship between students and teachers' also advances the view of educational environments as strictly hierarchical and to be tightly controlled by those in positions of authority, with punishment to be meted out for deviance from the norm. This is not an environment in which students who vary significantly from their peers in terms of behavior, cognition, social interaction, and support needs can expect to easily succeed.

Indeed, conformity of thought and behavior are key expectations in higher education in a number of ways, disadvantaging many of those with diverse needs that do not fit within the narrow acceptable range. Brown and Leigh (2020) point to how 'academic ecosystems seek to normalise and homogenise ways of working and being a scholar' (p. 5), and the pressures that increasingly corporatized higher education institutions experience to produce successful students en masse, making their individual differences a liability rather than a consideration (p. 3). Price (2011) argues that academia's valorization of a specific definition of 'rationality' makes it inherently hostile to different modes of thought and perception, including those of psychiatric and other disabilities affecting the mind (p. 8). Bolt and Penketh (2016) also collect a variety of scholarship highlighting the ways in which scholarship tends to avoid and dismiss the subject of disability altogether.

While higher education institutions have in recent years increasingly come to profess commitment to 'diversity, equity, and inclusion,' the vast majority simultaneously have not adequately reckoned with the rigid, normative, implicit expectations that academic structures, systems, facilities, and timelines impose on students (not to mention faculty), and tend to resist change to these whenever the possibility arises. Where this is true, the 'diversity' that an institution seeks can only be cosmetic in nature, only 'including' students from diverse backgrounds who are most able to perform the often grueling contortions of resembling those with privileged identities in how they think, speak, behave, and work, in order to be successful—and as long as this is the case, genuine equity will remain impossible.

Furthermore, another, particularly dismaying factor becomes evident in disabled students' narratives of their own experiences, as will become evident throughout this book: these expectations of conformity are, more often than not, shared by the students themselves, and their difficulties in meeting them are perceived as their own personal failings. Internalized ableism and its attendant negative self-perceptions, as Charlton (1998) puts it, 'prevent people with disabilities from knowing their real selves, their real needs, and their real capabilities and from recognizing the options they in fact have' (p. 27). So, too, do students who have been told there is something wrong with them enough times come to believe it, and that it is reasonable to expect them to conform to the expectations set for people very different from them, without adjustment, material support, or any but superficial accommodations.

Capacity Challenges

At the individual level, however, while support for students with disabilities is, indeed, lacking in higher education, this is often not out of any lack of desire by staff and faculty to help. Rather, even those who want to provide sufficient services for neurodivergent and disabled students are frequently unable to do so. Improved diagnosis and increased access to higher education have led in recent decades to rapidly burgeoning populations of disabled students, especially those who are neurodivergent or have other cognitive, emotional, and behavioral differences (Madaus, 2011, pp. 11–12). While in many ways this is a positive development, and ideally institutions would embrace transformative change to meet the challenge of this new student diversity, in practice this transformation has mostly failed to materialize. This leaves disability services staff, as well as other staff and faculty who want to support neurodivergent and disabled students, to be overwhelmed with new needs while not receiving commensurate increases in resources, support, or staffing, and without substantial changes to university structures and policies that unfairly hinder these students and restrict what even the best-intentioned employees can do for them.

These issues have been exacerbated by the legislative rollback that Madaus (2011) notes has occurred since ADA's passage, where a number of court cases have effectively led to curtailment of its reach and impact. Among other things, this backlash and its results have played a role in preventing a systematic, accountable approach to implementing ADA in higher education. While some institutions have been more successful in embracing disability support in a holistic, collaborative way, no consistency has been supported or enforced, and many more institutions have been unsuccessful. On most campuses, knowledge of and support for disabilities is piecemeal and inconsistently available, limited to individual sympathetic staff and faculty members scattered across departments, meaning that the onus falls on disabled and neurodivergent students to disclose information about their needs and try to uncover support where it can be found (Kershbaum et al., 2017, pp. 1–2). As Charlton (1998) also notes, furthermore, there is a material cost for full access to inaccessible public spaces like colleges and universities for people with disabilities, and governing bodies have been as reluctant to fund those costs and facilitate structures of access in higher education as they seem to be in all other areas of public life in the U.S. (pp. 87–92). Higher education has in fact been perpetually underfunded in general in many states, and faculty and staff departments increasingly understaffed, undersupported, precariously employed, and stretched thin. Fewer economic and personal resources in general, of course, mean fewer that might be diverted to serving students with disabilities, or to any specific work toward equity.

A number of factors have contributed to this environment of relative scarcity in higher education. One significant cause, however, which also bears on other issues for students with disabilities, is the growing influence of neoliberalism in the political environment.

Neoliberalism and Academic Capitalism

In the introduction to the blistering *Neoliberalism's War on Higher Education*, Giroux (2014) defines neoliberalism in excoriating terms: as an increasingly prevalent attitude of 'economic Darwinism,' eschewing values of public good and social responsibility in favor of individualistic gain. As Giroux describes it, neoliberalism views all success and failure as a matter of individual worth, meaning that it habitually ignores existing systemic, societal inequities that face marginalized communities. This means, in turn, that these inequities remain in place and go unchallenged, and continue to privilege the privileged and marginalize the marginalized, reinforcing existing disparities. The effects are only exacerbated by neoliberalism's 'expansion of a punishing state that increasingly criminalizes a range of social behaviors, wages war on the poor instead of poverty, militarizes local police forces, harasses poor minority youth, and spends more on prisons than on higher education' (Giroux, 2014, p. 22). It is a political ideology that, as Giroux ultimately condemns it, is implemented by plutocrats in order to uphold plutocracy, and is characterized by cruelty, lack of compassion, and apathy toward the ethical.

As a marginalized person with a commitment to social justice and a scholar of the humanities, who has closely observed the political developments of the United States in the past decades, I find I cannot disagree with Giroux's assessment, either of the nature of neoliberalism or of its increasing influence. Neither can I refute Giroux's identification of the impacts that this environment has on higher education. One of these has been a push, in part imposed from the state level upon higher education institutions, to target the curriculum increasingly toward career training, and away from critical thinking and engagement with moral issues (Giroux, 2014). For examples, one need only look to recent headlines describing attempted bans on critical engagement with racial inequality in education, or bills in Florida to eliminate DEI initiatives from higher education altogether. Another has been the rise of academic capitalism, defined by Slaughter and Leslie (1997) as the reorientation of scholarship and knowledge production toward a profit motive. Funding cuts and increasing suspicion toward educational institutions as a public good have plagued colleges and universities under the influence of neoliberalism, and have played a part in pushing them to pursue business-influenced models and sources of financial gain in order to sustain themselves. This is a shift that critics like Giroux feel fundamentally undermines their intended purpose, as well as placing more of the expected financial burden of higher education on students themselves. Furthermore, as Slaughter and Rhoades (2004) note, this shift demonstrably decreases the quality of services in higher education and makes knowledge itself a more privatized, corporate product, while also not actually generating much in the way of profit—at least not for academic institutions (pp. 330–332). Instead, it funnels the investments that are made into nonprofit higher education away to private corporate profits, for university trustees' private businesses and other new partners in the for-profit sector (Slaughter, 2014, pp. 24–25).

As a result, the influence of neoliberalism on higher education has negative impacts for all students, but there are factors that are of significance for students with disabilities in particular. One of these is what Giroux (2014) refers to as the 'politics of disposability' (p. 12): a willingness to abandon the marginalized to the forces that oppress them, and to blame them for failing to succeed under these conditions. If, under academic capitalism, all students are considered consumers and revenue streams, then the material costs needed to make education accessible for disabled students offset their potential profits, and therefore make these students less desirable than others. No matter how the institution may claim to want to serve a diverse student body, as long as it is a priority for students to represent a financial return on investment, it will not be considered in the best interests of the institution to take on and retain students who require more than minimal support to succeed.

Another factor particularly affecting disabled students is how faculty are affected by the neoliberal university. Academic capitalism tends to lead toward expansion of managerial power and an increased proportion of nonacademic staff (Slaughter, 2014, p. 13), which leads in turn to erosion of faculty power in institutional governance, demoralizing them and often resulting in negative trends in their working conditions (Giroux, 2014). Particularly in universities, administration has increasingly found it more cost-effective to reduce tenure lines, and delegate an increasing amount of instruction to non-tenure-track faculty, adjunct faculty, graduate students, and other contingent or contracted employees. On the whole, these instructors are overworked, undercompensated, unbenefited, and precariously employed, making for an overall faculty that is much less willing and able to take academic risks or work beyond minimum requirements for instruction—as well as straining the remaining tenure-track faculty, as they scramble to cover duties that can only be completed by those in their role. It is quite reasonable that faculty in this position are less willing and able to support any of their students in meaningful ways, let alone their students with unique needs. Creating accessible course environments, fully supporting students with accommodations, being flexible with timelines, and other adjustments badly needed by disabled students are all critical tasks that nonetheless take work, and as most institutions have not made provisions for that work at a systemic level, it falls on the individual course faculty to decide whether or not to complete it. When already overextended, under-resourced, and in many cases completely without job security or benefits, it is less likely than ever that faculty will choose to undertake these extra tasks, even if their attitudes toward students with disabilities are more positive than average.

Specific Stigma around Learning and Psychiatric Disabilities

Finally, and more specifically of concern for the types of disabilities under discussion here, students perceived as having learning disabilities or psychiatric conditions are in many ways particularly at risk of stigma in higher education, over students with other types of disabilities. As Oslund (2014) describes, a number of myths about students with invisible disabilities pervade higher education, such as that an anxiety disorder is no worse than the type of nervousness everyone experiences in academic situations and can be overcome with continued exposure, or that accommodations can represent unfair advantages, or that invisible disabilities are easily faked or overdiagnosed. Many of these myths, as Oslund also acknowledges, stem from simple lack of familiarity with the conditions in question. Similarly, faculty may also assume that rigor must be compromised for students with learning disabilities to succeed, imagining that 'learning disabilities' indicate that these students are less able to do academic work—rather than understanding that they only have more difficulty with the traditional mechanics of the work.

Experiencing challenges with certain modes of taking in information or demonstrating learning, however, does not make a student any less capable of actual learning.

Students with psychiatric disabilities, meanwhile, face an even more complex set of stigmatizing and disabling factors in college. In part this is simply because psychiatric disabilities tend to be heavily stigmatized in general: when discussing the 'hierarchy of disability,' Charlton (1998) notes that mental illness tends to be relegated to the bottom, with the mentally ill most subject to stigma, ostracization, and harm across cultures (p. 97). Furthermore, in the 2011 *Mad at School: Rhetorics of Mental Disability and Academic Life,* Price provides a powerful overview of the uneasy ways that mental disability chafes against the expectations of academia in particular, for mentally disabled students and faculty. These include scholarly valorization of 'rationality' and homogeneity of ways of thinking and reasoning (pp. 8–9), and the flawed but ubiquitous association of 'mental illness' with acts of school violence, which creates a perceived need to protect educational institutions from mentally ill students, rather than the other way around (pp. 142–144). Furthermore, academic and other forms of stress have recently been driving a growing crisis in the need for campus mental health care, for students with preexisting mental health conditions and those without, which available counseling resources have proven insufficient to meet (Abrams, 2022). Even students with mental health needs who are aware of those needs and able to reach out for help—which, as later chapters will show, already represent a minority—may not be able to access resources on campus to help them.

Summary and Conclusions

Higher education has a long history of being a hostile landscape for people with disabilities in general. Over time, however, activists in a number of social movements have pushed to create spaces for disabled students in colleges and universities: Deaf students, disabled veterans, proponents of the independent living movement, and advocates for legislative reform have all contributed to this work, among others. Their efforts have helped make college success more attainable for disabled students, although in ways frequently complicated by issues of race, gender, class, and other factors, and not without lingering barriers that still plague students today. These include the implicit expectations, norms, hierarchies, and carceral attitudes embedded in higher education systems. They also include limitations in the human and financial resources available to support disabled students, which have been increasingly imposed by the growing influence of neoliberalism on public life in the U.S. Neoliberalism has also impacted higher education in other ways that are to the detriment of disabled students' success, such as causing 'less profitable' students with greater support needs to be considered less desirable, and placing increasing strain on faculty that makes it less possible for them to adequately support students with disabilities. All of these issues are only compounded for students with conditions classified as learning disabilities and psychiatric disabilities, who face additional stigma and challenges in higher education institutions because of stereotypes and misperceptions about what their conditions imply. Understanding all of these inherent factors and how they impact neurodivergent and disabled college students will be critical to contextualizing the experiences that students have recounted in the research literature.

2. Terminology, Categories, and Complicating Factors

Choices of language and construction of categories are always significant when discussing marginalized communities, and perhaps especially so when it comes to neurodiversity and disability. How one rhetorically organizes and refers to disabled people reflects one's own attitudes and understandings at least as much as it does the practical facts of bodies and minds. The 'correct' language is seldom a settled matter, furthermore, and valid arguments can be made for a variety of rhetorical approaches to these complex subjects. Often more important than the individual rhetorical choices is making those choices intentionally, thoughtfully, and explicitly.

Toward this end, this chapter will attempt to comprehensively define the categories and terms that will be in use throughout the remainder of this book. I will explain the ways I have chosen to organize and describe the identities of those I am here calling 'neurodivergent and invisibly disabled students,' and also why these choices are appropriate for my purposes. My framings should not be understood to represent definitive constructions or terminologies for any of the categories in question. They are simply those I have found best suited to the work of this book, and certainly neither without flaws nor necessarily suitable for other contexts. In fact, another element I will discuss as I review my framework will be its limitations, and how the practical realities of students' identities are certain to be far more complex and nuanced than what I am able to describe here.

　　https://doi.org/10.11647/OBP.0420.02

Categories Under Consideration

When I say this book is about the experiences of 'neurodivergent and invisibly disabled students,' to whom am I referring? This is admittedly a slightly cumbersome label, though I felt that was necessary to be as accurate and nuanced as possible, but it is still not an unambiguous one. For my purposes here, this label should be understood to include students in six rough categories of conditions, whose experiences I have examined by category and across categories. These conditions are:

1. Dyslexia and related conditions

2. Attention deficit hyperactivity disorder (ADHD)

3. Autism

4. Psychiatric disabilities

5. Traumatic brain injuries (TBI)

6. Disabling chronic physical illnesses

A more extended discussion of how I define each of these categories follows.

Dyslexia and Related Conditions

This category focuses specifically on students with reading, writing, and other lexical challenges that affect their studies. As Oslund (2014) notes, this category is somewhat mislabeled: 'In every day usage, people tend to refer to all language disorders as "dyslexia." While dyslexia is one language disorder, technically, not all language disorders are dyslexia' (p. 68). For the purpose of this work, however, I have followed the everyday usage, primarily because the label of 'dyslexia' tends to be applied to all research studies about students with language disorders, regardless of its complete accuracy. Furthermore, the 'related conditions' mentioned include dysgraphia (specific writing challenges), dyscalculia (specific mathematical challenges), and dyspraxia (specific physical coordination challenges) under this umbrella. While not all of these disabilities are alike, and those that are not 'dyslexia' proper are disabling in educational contexts in specific and unique ways, unfortunately none of the rest have been substantively and separately studied in this context, while dyslexia has. Where they appear in the literature, therefore, I have associated them with the broad 'dyslexia' label because of the taxonomical similarities, while recognizing that this is an imperfect grouping.

ADHD

This category focuses on students who have attention, concentration, memory, and executive function challenges in a higher education context. As noted in Oslund (2014), the specific symptoms and diagnostic criteria for ADHD are particularly complex, which may be compounded by the tendency of ADHD characteristics to shift and evolve over the lifetime of a person with the condition (Shea et al., 2019, p. 20). Hyperactivity, in particular, may tend to be less of an issue for many students by the time they reach college age. The primary unifying theme in ADHD symptoms, in any case, seems to be difficulty with self-regulation (Shea et al., 2019, p. 20). In literature studying student experiences, furthermore, there is a tendency to collapse students with ADHD into other categories of students with learning disabilities, often to the point of using 'ADHD' and 'learning disabilities' interchangeably. This leads into some ambiguities in what are considered characteristics of students with ADHD, as well as some conflation of ADHD symptoms with those that may more accurately be of dyslexia and related conditions. This ambiguity is made both more understandable and more challenging by the fact that there tends to be significant overlap in the symptoms of ADHD and dyslexia, as well as co-occurrence of the two conditions in the same student. These first two categories will therefore often be discussed in conjunction as student experiences are addressed in later chapters.

Autism

I have used the category of 'autism' to broadly encompass all types of expression along the autism spectrum. This means that there is sometimes wide variation in the literature between different students in this category, as by this definition, autistic students may be very different from one another in terms of their behaviors and characteristics. What they are most likely to share in common are challenges in social interaction and relationships, idiosyncratic and repeating behaviors, need for routine and predictability, particular sensitivity to sensory input, and intense focus on particular subjects. It should also be noted that a few terms appear frequently in the literature under study that I choose not to use. One of these is that some studies here refer to Asperger's Disorder (or similar phrasings), as they were published prior to the 2013 removal of Asperger's Disorder from the DSM and reorganization under Autism Spectrum Disorder. Another, however, is that I choose to reject the language of 'high-functioning' and 'low-functioning' autism. As many autistic advocates have noted, these labels prioritize facility in certain areas according to the biases of a neurotypical perspective, and create an unnecessary hierarchization of autistic characteristics and behaviors, while not actually providing meaningful information about where the autistic person in question has facility or needs support, nor recognizing that appropriate support may help them succeed regardless of inherent characteristics (ASAN, 2021). Even where studies have identified student participants using these terms, therefore, I have eschewed them, in favor of specifying characteristics where possible.

Psychiatric Disabilities

This is the term that will be used to encompass mental health disorders, mental illness, and similar chronic or acute illnesses affecting thought, emotions, and behavior. Choice of terminology in this category can be particularly loaded, as Price (2011) acknowledges in the introduction to *Mad at School*, before articulating a rationale for using the term 'mental disability' in that work: to encourage broadness of definition and invite coalition between those with various types of disability that exist within the mind. I greatly respect and appreciate Price's thoughtful choice of 'mental disability' for those purposes, even as I choose 'psychiatric disabilities' for mine: to match the language most commonly used in the research I examine to describe this population. After all, more categories in this work than this one could be referred to as 'mental disabilities,' and here it will be helpful to be more specific to contrast with those, even when there is also significant overlap between categories. 'Psychiatric disabilities' is the term I found to recur most often in research studies when referring to the types of conditions in this category, and even those that did not use it tended to use terms ('mental illness,' 'mental health disorders,' etc.) with a similar connotation of disease in need of medical treatment. This is not necessarily correct or incorrect as a rhetorical framing, but it is one that I find worth explicitly recognizing. In any case, by far the most commonly occurring conditions in this category, in the literature and typically in general, are anxiety and depression. A few studies, however, also deal with students living with others, such as post-traumatic stress disorder or psychosis.

Traumatic Brain Injuries (TBI)

This category deals with students who have experienced a physical injury to the brain that has caused disabling changes in thinking and cognition, motor coordination, emotion, behavior, or day-to-day-functioning, or combinations of any of these. While there are relatively few studies specifically on students with TBI, they are somewhat more often included in broader studies of students with multiple types of invisible disabilities. This is also arguably one of the categories with the most variation in form, presentation, and impact, leading sometimes to inconsistent conclusions between and even within research studies.

Disabling Chronic Physical Illness

While I will refer to this category simply as 'chronic illness' for the most part in the text, some qualification is useful at this definitional stage. Here I am referring specifically to chronic illness that is physical in nature, to distinguish it from other types of chronic illness, which fall under other categories in this work. I am also referring specifically to chronic illness that is disabling, to distinguish it from minor conditions that may be experienced in the long term but do not significantly impact day-to-day life activities. Those conditions still encompass a very wide variety of individual impairments, making this in many ways a slippery category with elusive boundaries. In general, I have chosen only to include conditions that cannot inherently or normally be perceived by an outside observer, and that cause a significant impact to the student's life, based on self-descriptions in the relevant studies. As with TBI, however, these criteria for inclusion have occasionally resulted in a widely varying set of presentations and conclusions.

Why These, and Why Not Others?

Of the top ten types of disabilities in students aged three through twenty-one served by IDEA, I would describe six as most likely to go unnoticed by the average external observer: specific learning disability, health impairment, autism, development delay, intellectual disability, and emotional disturbance (National Center for Education Statistics, 2023). The categories I have chosen here are what I have found to be the most commonly occurring manifestations of these disability types in studies of college students' experiences: dyslexia and related conditions are most common in terms of learning disabilities, ADHD may be classed as a learning or an intellectual disability, and traumatic brain injuries may cause symptoms that span a number of these disability types. While not all of the studies that I have examined have used these exact terms to describe their studied populations, they have all fallen into these rough categories.

Of course, this is not a comprehensive list of all invisible disabilities and neurodiversity. Visual, hearing, and mobility disabilities, for example, may also affect college students in ways that are not obvious to an outside observer. These types of disability, however, are more likely to at least affect the student's interactions with the environment in visible ways. The same is true of conditions like epilepsy, and other physical and neurological illnesses that were not included within the scope of my research. They are also less common in this age group than those that I have listed, as the NCES data shows. For my purposes here, I was interested in the specific experiences of students with a physical or mental difference that cannot be readily observed by others, and that therefore may be treated with doubt, skepticism, and lack of understanding by others, in ways that compound barriers and make supports more challenging to obtain. I was also forced to exclude some types of neurodivergence and disability—Tourette syndrome, for one notable example—simply because sufficient research had not been conducted on the experiences of students with those types of conditions. Hopefully this limitation will be removed as research continues in this area.

It is also worth noting that, in many ways, chronic illness seems like the odd category out in my chosen list. It is the only type of disability listed that does not necessarily relate to cognition, for one thing, and for another, though it is still more likely to be invisible than not, it is more likely to manifest in externally visible ways than are the others. Indeed, initially I only included chronic illness in my research out of personal interest, due to my own experiences in this area. Once I had begun to explore student experiences with chronic illness, however, I found that the population of chronically ill students significantly overlaps with the other categories I was studying, and that similar inherent issues and patterns are shared across the experiences of chronically ill students and the students in the other categories. Based on my observations, I have come to believe that chronic illness should be examined alongside disabilities relating to cognition, emotion, and behavior, if only for these reasons.

Why these Labels for the Categories?

Admittedly, the terms that I have chosen to define each of these categories tend toward medicalized diagnostic labels, which is potentially problematic. Classifying students' experiences in this way can tread in the territory of what Linton (1998) has called 'medical meaning-making,' or imposing narratives of medical impairment and rehabilitation on disabled people's experiences even when it is not appropriate. Indeed, many of the studies I have examined do not even internally use these labels to describe the students who were interviewed, even when I have classified them according to these terms for the purposes of my work. Hollins and Foley (2013), for example, classify the self-descriptions of their participants by the impact of the impairment(s) on each student's learning, which I found to be a thoughtfully nuanced and possibly more helpful approach for their purposes.

In my case, however, my system of organization has its basis in my methodology, which was a review of the literature. As a librarian, I am uniquely equipped with the skillset for this research approach, but I am also acutely aware of some of the more problematic aspects of a literature search on a topic like this, and one such aspect is the use of controlled vocabulary. In the organization of information, a controlled vocabulary is a set of terms that are used to standardize the potentially disparate language that may be used to refer to a single topic, to facilitate more effective searching and browsing. For example, a controlled vocabulary might implement 'ADHD' as the term to be used over 'attention deficit hyperactivity disorder,' 'attention deficit disorder,' and similar terms when searching for the same concept. In searching for scholarly literature, this generally takes the form of subject terms and thesauri within library databases, which can be used to help select appropriate, relevant search terms for the desired results. When searching, I used controlled vocabulary terms to guide my choices of language for each category. The main exception was the case of psychiatric disabilities, where I needed to employ a variety of possible terms, but even then I ultimately chose to name the category for the descriptor used in common by the greatest majority of studies.

Controlled vocabularies, however, are necessarily human-generated and particularly laborious to produce and maintain. Because of these factors, and because of the wide range of perspectives on a topic they must serve, they tend to be conservative in their choices of terms, and slow to adapt to social-justice-oriented shifts in language on sensitive topics relating to marginalized communities. True to form, the standard subject terms in use for the types of difference I chose to study reflect a medicalized, regimented construction of types of neurodivergence and invisible disability, which many activists and advocates would find outdated, if not outright oppressive. Nevertheless, these were the terms that were applied to the studies that I wished to locate, and that I therefore needed to use to retrieve that information. As a result, I label my categories roughly according to the vocabulary that I mainly used to conduct my literature search, both for the sake of accuracy and to implicitly acknowledge the limitations imposed by my research medium.

Problems of Defining Categories

As tidy as these categories may appear on paper, furthermore, in the actual lives of students the truth is always much more complex. While such labels are helpful in organizing and understanding the available information, they are not without their problems in application to lived experience. One significant problem is that defining these categories this way implies that each of these conditions exists as a binary system: either a student 'has ADHD' or 'is chronically ill,' definitively and completely and in all respects, or does not and is not. This is a general understanding of disability and neurodivergence, in fact, that is as prevalent as it is overly simplistic. The reality is that each of these categories in some way represents a continuum, as Fletcher et al. (2018) explain with regard to learning disabilities, along which cutoff points or boundaries have to be artificially imposed to determine what constitutes 'disabled' on one side, and 'not disabled' on the other (pp. 35–36). This will, of course, always be a source of intense discomfort for those closest to that cutoff line, from either side. Many students who would be diagnosed as nondisabled or neurotypical may have one or more significant disabled or neurodivergent traits, just not to the same degree or in the same quantity as students diagnosed as disabled or neurodivergent. The reverse is also true: some students who would be diagnosed as disabled or neurodivergent by standard criteria nonetheless may not be significantly impacted by some of the classic traits associated with that diagnosis. People who fit into these categories are not of another species; the characteristics that affect their lives are part of the complete range of variation in human minds and bodies, and those variations show up in many forms and degrees, within and without the imposed boundaries of what constitutes a disability. This is not at all to suggest, however, that students in these categories do not need or deserve supports to help them be successful, or that they are not truly disadvantaged or discriminated against in education, or that their differences are insignificant because 'everyone feels that way sometimes.' On the contrary, it is to suggest that far more students could benefit from supports, flexibility, and increased accessibility than just those who receive formal diagnoses in these categories, and that the common gatekeeping idea that only certain students are 'disabled enough' to 'deserve' supports and accommodations is fundamentally flawed.

This is particularly true because not nearly all students who *could* be diagnosed with these conditions *are* diagnosed—or share their diagnosis with their educational institutions, even if they are. As will be discussed in detail in later chapters, one of the single biggest problems in supporting invisibly disabled and neurodivergent students is how commonly they are diagnosed late in life, not diagnosed at all, alienated from their diagnosis, determined not to seek support in spite of it, or some combination of these. Even when a student, their parents, and their teachers may suspect the student is disabled or neurodivergent, obtaining a formal diagnosis is often a costly process in time and money in itself, and not necessarily available to all. Furthermore, by their inherent nature, invisible disabilities are easily overlooked, both by others and by students themselves, who have no basis for comparison for their internal experiences. Especially with disabilities that affect learning and cognition, students may assume that their struggles are universal and must simply be overcome, or internalize others' harmful and ill-informed accusations of laziness, underachievement, and lack of capacity for learning. Conditions in these categories may also vary widely enough in presentation that students with atypical symptoms may have difficulty being accurately diagnosed simply because they defy typical categorization.

Even when formally diagnosed, students may continue to doubt and blame themselves, or feel that they do not 'count' as disabled, or believe that they do not 'deserve' support. They may also resist asking for help for a variety of rational reasons, such as fear of stigma when they disclose negatively stereotyped conditions, or lack of time to navigate the bureaucracy of receiving accommodations, or lack of confidence that the available supports will be helpful even if they are obtained. Because of the uniquely malleable nature of disability, personal identification as disabled can be complex, precarious, and conditional with any type of impairment, as noted by Siebers (2016, pp. 4–6) among others. This is doubly true in those with invisible disabilities, as they do not fit the common expectation of what disability looks like. Alienation from the idea of being disabled is also, necessarily, alienation from the idea of having accessibility needs, and makes these students less likely to seek out explanations or adjustments for difficulties in learning that they may not realize are excessive.

A final factor that complicates the categories I have listed here, also, is that they are by no means as discrete from one another as my description so far has implied. As will also become apparent in later chapters, there is significant overlap and permeability between many of the categories under discussion here, where characteristics of one may not be readily distinguishable from those of another. There is also, similarly, a great deal of co-occurrence of these categories—to the point that I have found it to be more common for any given student interviewed in a research study to fit more than one of these categories than to fit only one. Some degree of psychiatric disability, in particular, is extremely likely to coexist with a disability or neurodivergence in any of the other categories, in some cases related to the other condition and in some not. This intertwining of these categories is one of the strongest reasons that I find it most logical to examine them all as a group, rather than focusing on only one or a smaller grouping.

Choices of Terminology

'Neurodivergent and invisibly disabled'

As mentioned near the beginning of this chapter, I have chosen the term 'neurodivergent and invisibly disabled' (and similar permutations) to refer to the entire population under discussion in this book, in spite of the clumsiness of the term. The obvious question would be why I do not simply say 'invisibly disabled,' if I am already defining this term in a specific way that admittedly does exclude some recognized forms of invisible disability. Some neurodivergent people might even refer to themselves as having an invisible disability. The main reason that I have chosen to use both terms, however, is that others would not identify as having a disability—even if they would identify as disabled. The distinction between the two points to a gap between different rhetorical framings of what being 'disabled' means.

The neurodiversity paradigm, which has been embraced by many activists for the civil rights of neurodivergent people, positions neurotypicality and various forms of neurodivergence as value-neutral variations in modes of human thought and behavior. It also rejects pathologizing terminology like 'disorder' to refer to neurodivergence, and prioritizes happy and healthy lives for neurodivergent people, and not 'curing' or otherwise eliminating neurodivergence. Silberman (2015), for example, uses the metaphor of computer operating systems to explain the framing, in the sense that two systems may run in quite different ways but neither is broken (p. 471). There have been critiques of the neurodiversity paradigm, claiming that it fails to adequately recognize that some neurodivergent people struggle with major difficulties because of their conditions, and that it gives outsized power to those most able to communicate and advocate in neurotypical-like ways (Russell, 2019, pp. 293–294). I and many neurodiversity advocates would argue, however, that it is instead having to operate within a neurotypically-dominated society that gives the advantage to certain neurodivergent voices, not the nature of the movement itself. Furthermore, framing neurodivergence as value-neutral does not mean that it presents no difficulties for neurodivergent people that need to be addressed. Rather, neurodiversity advocacy positions those difficulties with the biases and oppression of dominant neurotypical culture, rather than within neurodivergent people themselves. This is the crux of the distinction between 'having a disability' and 'disabled' mentioned above. As Walker (2021) frames this distinction:

> To say 'autism is a disability' is to perpetuate the frameworks of the pathology paradigm and the medical model of disability, by framing autism as a problem located within the autistic individual. To say 'autistic people are disabled,' by contrast, embraces the frameworks of the neurodiversity paradigm and the social model of disability—and opens the door to better approaches to autistic well-being—by framing autistic disablement as being the result of correctible mismatches between autistic needs and societal accommodations. (pp. 65–66)

In this framing, while the neurodivergent person does indeed experience hardship arising from their condition, that hardship is the result of navigating an environment not suited to them, not evidence that their condition is a disease to be cured.

   This is not to say, however, that critiques of the neurodiversity paradigm are not substantive, nor that this is the only one. Much of the advocacy for the paradigm has been from white neurodivergent activists, for example, and DisCrit and other critiques of color of the paradigm have begun to emerge, pointing to the white-centrism of many of its constructions and priorities (Kofke & Krazinski, 2024); for one example, the serious risks of police violence that face Black autistic men deserve urgent attention and work and have yet to be prioritized by most research (Hutson et al., 2022). In theory, the neurodiversity paradigm is not by any means exclusive of addressing key intersectional concerns, but in practice its focus has a tendency to skew white, simply because of the whiteness of who is likely to self-identify and be identified as neurodivergent (as will be discussed in more detail in Chapter 6). There are also questions to be raised as to whether the specialized framing of 'neurodiversity' constitutes a form of stratification and lateral ableism, attempting to elevate and valorize one type of disability by declining to associate it with the label of 'disability' at all, and meanwhile tacitly conceding the framing of disability as inherently negative—not entirely dissimilar from the historical moves of the Deaf community described in Chapter 1. These concerns should be acknowledged and are worth considering. Nonetheless, given the embrace of the neurodiversity paradigm by the most prominent liberatory activists in this area and the positive aspects it does offer, I have chosen to make use of the term 'neurodivergent' in this context, albeit with caveats.

As Walker mentions in the quotation above, for example, the neurodiversity paradigm aligns with the social model of disability, which was developed to support advocacy for the rights of disabled people, in opposition to the medical model's focus on repairing perceived individual faults (Oliver, 1983). Shea et al. (2019) acknowledge the extension of this model into a social justice model, which focuses on the ways that disabled people are marginalized and how ableism pervades social systems, and recognizes the ways that being disabled may intersect with other marginalized identities (pp. 6–7). Gleeson (1998) also notes how this model has been deepened by theorists, including Oliver (1996), to describe disability as 'both a socially and historically relative identity that is *produced* [author's emphasis] by society' (p. 25). To perhaps oversimplify, what constitutes being disabled is contextual and linked to the norms and expectations of one's culture, and a person who is positioned as disabled in one context might not be so in another. Among other things, these framings help to clarify why disability is so difficult to concretely define: like race, rather than an empirical, biological fact, it can instead be understood as a category of marginalization, constructed by perceptions, culture, and systems in its local context.

Under this definition, as Walker (2021) also recognizes, not all neurodivergent people are disabled. Within the overlapping cultural contexts of the United States, of the West, and of higher education, there are certainly college students who I would classify as neurodivergent who nonetheless are not meaningfully disabled by the systems and perceptions around them. Even so, however, these students may have unique experiences and even hardships in higher education that are worth noting alongside those of their disabled peers. There are also neurodivergent students who are disabled, and there are also of course invisibly disabled students considered here who I would not classify as neurodivergent. For these reasons, I have chosen to include both of these overlapping categories when referring to my complete population in the interest of greatest accuracy, with the acknowledgment that sometimes both terms are referring to the same set of people, and other times not.

Person-First vs. Identity-First Language

Walker's framing of disability also highlights another contentious element of terminology, which is the choice of whether to use person-first or identity-first language. That is to say, whether to refer to 'people with disabilities' (person-first) or 'disabled people' (identity-first). Many official and professional settings, such as the American Psychological Association for example, have adopted and recommend person-first language. This serves the stated purpose of foregrounding the humanity of people with disabilities, an important response to the frequently dehumanizing history and present of disability rights, and also indicating that an impairment does not define the whole of a person. Disability rights advocates like Walker, however, contest this language for the reasons stated, out of the rhetorical framing of the social model of disability: that this language still positions a 'disability' as a fault located in the individual, and it is preferable to emphasize the 'disablement' that results from systemic failures and oppression of those with an impairment. Scholarship in disability studies has also often chosen to adopt this language for the same reasons, such as in the example of Gleeson (1998). As Shea et al. (2019) point out, however, some controversy over the terms still remains.

My personal conclusion has been that both terms have something to offer in terms of their rhetorical focus, but in most cases I do prefer to use identify-first language in this book, because my goal is to address the social justice issue of how higher education environments are disabling. In particular, I have chosen to use only identify-first language when referring to neurodivergent people and especially autistic people, as a particularly strong consensus has formed among advocates for these communities rejecting person-first language (Sinclair, 1999; Walker, 2021).

When referring to invisible disabilities more broadly, however, I have chosen to follow the professional recommendation of some psychologists to use both configurations of language (Dunn & Andrews, 2015). I vary between person-first and identity-first language throughout the text, and this is not an inadvertent inconsistency but an intentional choice. In so doing, I intend to recognize that while ableist environments and systems are indeed disabling in all cases, many invisibly disabled people *do* also experience disability as an intrinsic and unwelcome burden, from which they might prefer to be rhetorically distanced. Price (2011) acknowledges tension between the disability advocacy model and the experiences of some people with mental disabilities (pp. 12–13), for example, and Wendell (2001) discusses how disability advocacy has often framed disability in ways that exclude people with chronic illnesses.

Furthermore, I am guided by my own perspective as an invisibly disabled person, in which I personally experience suffering that is inherent to the nature of my disabling conditions, as well as suffering that is imposed from without by ableist systems, environments, and expectations—even while I recognize that this is not the experience of all disabled people, particularly not those that Wendell (2001) refers to as the 'healthy disabled.' For me, my conditions simply are not benign variations in possible ways of being, nor even necessarily identities that make me who I am, and I would not be entirely at ease with their being framed that way. They are medical conditions and, while they cannot be 'cured,' they require medical treatment for the sake of my quality of life. At the same time, there are many disabled people who feel just the opposite, and rightly resist the framing of their differences as medical disorders in need of 'curing' (i.e. elimination). Both perspectives are valid, and both belong to people who share the identity of 'disabled,' even while they represent a major divide within that category. It is nonetheless necessary, however, for us to reach across that divide for the sake of our coalition, if for no other reason than because the boundaries within our community are too blurry for us to do otherwise. Is a person with multiple sclerosis or cerebral palsy, for example, more 'disabled' or more 'ill'? For that matter, should every condition that causes suffering in itself be ousted from the category of the disabled, and further splinter a marginalized community already struggling to secure our rights?

It is in recognition of these ambiguities and points of contention that I use only identity-first language for neurodivergent people, but alternate between identity-first and person-first for invisibly disabled people in general. While I recognize that this is an imperfect way of capturing all of the nuance encompassed by these broad labels, it represents my best attempt to acknowledge in a concise phrase the many variations in experience within the conditions under discussion.

Summary and Conclusions

Many complex issues of identity, marginalization, and equity surround any discussion of disabled and neurodivergent students, and these demand care in how we handle language and categorization. With this in mind, I have chosen to identify and categorize the populations under discussion in this book as follows: dyslexic students and those with related conditions, students with ADHD, autistic students, students with psychiatric disabilities, students with traumatic brain injuries, and students with disabling chronic physical illnesses. I chose to use this language because it corresponds to the language used in searching the literature in my research, and I chose these categories because they represent the conditions most likely to invisibly affect the lives of students in my target demographic. At the same time, I also recognize that whether or not a student belongs to one of these categories is in reality a much more complex and nuanced issue than this categorization makes it appear.

I am also mindful of the contextual meaning of the word 'disabled,' and how the social model of disability encourages a view of disablement as a marginalized identity created by social context, rather than necessarily a fact originating from within the body. I have chosen to use the term 'neurodivergent and invisibly disabled' to refer to my entire population, to acknowledge that the students whose experiences I have studied represent two overlapping but distinct categories, and to recognize that one is not always the other even when the two may co-occur. Given prevailing sentiment among activists and advocates from these groups, I have also chosen to use only identity-first language when referring to neurodivergent people generally and to autistic people in particular. I vary between identity-first and person-first language for invisibly disabled people, however, to acknowledge that some do experience disablement as more internal, intrinsic, and debilitating. All of these intentional choices will be reflected throughout this book, as I discuss the experiences of different but overlapping populations.

PART II

CHALLENGES

3. Institutional Systems, Disability Services, and the Tensions of Self-Advocacy and Disclosure

Many of the current systems and structures of higher education can be fundamentally hostile to neurodivergent students and those with invisible disabilities. At minimum, these students may be required to make decisions and compromises in order to navigate their education that other students will not need to make, and they will likely need to learn additional strategies and coping mechanisms not required by their peers. Even though the most successful invisibly disabled and neurodivergent students may find long-term benefit from overcoming these additional challenges, they still represent inequities in the amount of effort different students must expend in order to achieve the same outcomes. In many cases, whether students are able to succeed in spite of more roadblocks is only a matter of chance and personality, rather than diligence or desire to learn. A student's success may also be directly hampered by the inherent characteristics of their difference. Even when university staff, faculty, and administrators have the best intentions of students at heart, the underlying assumptions and bureaucratic structures of the university still sometimes disproportionately set up certain students for failure.

Student outcomes show the impact of these inequities. According to the National Center for Education Statistics, the percentage of first-time students with disabilities who leave undergraduate education without return in their first year was 25.1% as of 2012, as opposed to 13.5% with no disability; 35.4% of students with disabilities had left without return by their second year, as opposed to 22.4% with no disability (United States Department of Education, 2017). Furthermore, not all disabilities

   https://doi.org/10.11647/OBP.0420.03

are reported, and students who are neurodivergent or have chronic illness, traumatic brain injury, or psychiatric disabilities tend to self-report at lower rates than other disability types. It is likely that some of the attrition assigned to students with 'no disability' in fact includes more students from these categories. Students with mental illness have been found to graduate at lower rates than those without—although their persistence rate appears to be comparable with that of students with other disability types (Salzer, 2012; Koch et al., 2014). Students with learning disabilities are also more likely to experience various types of barriers to their success in higher education, and to report lower overall satisfaction with their postsecondary experiences (McGregor et al., 2018).

With all of this in mind, this chapter will begin the discussion of the higher education experiences of neurodivergent and invisibly disabled students by providing an overview of their experiences with navigating higher education institutions overall, and the tensions they encounter in having to employ self-advocacy and disclosure of their conditions in order to do so. Foregrounded in the first area will be three types of experience that emerge as particularly relevant for these students:

1. Overall experiences, shared across multiple categories, that increase the challenges of participating in higher education;

2. Experiences with making decisions about institution and curriculum; and

3. Experiences interacting with and making use of institutional disability services offices.

It should be noted that disability services offices and personnel, in particular, are of tremendous importance to disabled students' overall higher education experiences. These resources serve as disabled students' primary means of making any necessary adaptations to their courses and learning environment, and thus students' experiences with them are likely to significantly impact their overall experiences. Relatedly, this chapter will also delve into the frequently conflicting desires and pressures students experience around disclosing neurodivergence and disabilities, asking for help, and advocating for their own needs to university faculty and staff. These, too, tend to fall into three main categories:

1. Reluctance to disclose and to seek help for needs, and the reasons behind this;

2. Issues around diagnosis and categorization of students, and the frequent requirement of documentation in order to qualify for accommodations; and

3. The role that disability identity plays in support-seeking, as well as why it may be problematic for many of the students under discussion here.

Between all of these elements, it should become evident why seeking supports is not a simple matter for neurodivergent students and those with invisible disabilities, and why true equity in higher education experiences may not be possible without drastic systemic reform.

Overall Challenges in Navigating Higher Education

One single most common challenge emerges from student narratives across all categories of neurodiversity and invisible disability. This is that significant additional burdens of time, labor, emotional distress, or all three are required to meet the same expectations that neurotypical and nondisabled students do. These extra burdens can take a number of different forms, depending on the typical characteristics and challenges of a category of difference. Multiple categories under discussion here tend to involve factors that directly affect the pace at which students can complete academic work, such as differences in cognition, reading, and other information processing that make reading and writing more laborious.[1] Difficulty concentrating is also a commonly reported symptom across multiple categories, whether this is inherent to the student's type of difference, or a result of distracting physical or psychiatric symptoms; this also extends the time required to complete independent assignments (Simmeborn Fleischer, 2012; Wennås Brante, 2013; Hong, 2015). Fatigue is another commonly recurring symptom, particularly

---

1   Bush et al., 2011; Erten, 2011; Melara, 2012; Mullins & Preyde, 2013; Wennås Brante, 2013; Downing, 2014; Kreider et al., 2015; Stampoltzis et al., 2015; Timmerman & Mulvihill, 2015; Childers & Hux, 2016; Hughes et al., 2016; Lefler, Sacchetti, & Del Carlo, 2016; Ward & Webster, 2018; James et al., 2020; Jones, 2020; Maurer-Smolder et al., 2021; Thompson, 2021.

given the commonality of sleep disturbances across these categories, and may cause delays and slow the pace at which students can complete academic work (Hughes et al., 2016). Academic schedules may also be in conflict with medical treatment schedules, especially for students with chronic illnesses, resulting in students being forced to choose between missing course deadlines or delaying treatment (Schwenk et al., 2014; Hoffman et al., 2019). Given all of these unavoidable factors interfering with their work, students with ADHD, in particular, often report the frustrating sense that they are investing tremendous time and effort into their studies, but their academic results are not commensurate with that effort or in line with their expectations of themselves (Hubbard, 2011; Young, 2012).

Outside of the academic curriculum, however, neurodivergent students and those with invisible disabilities face other disproportionate demands on their time and effort. Another activity into which students may need to invest these resources is advocating for their own needs in terms of disability support, and navigating the process of qualifying for and obtaining institutional accommodations (Strnadová et al., 2015; Lizotte, 2018). As Hollins and Foley (2013) point out, even if help is available to surmount barriers in the academic environment, having to seek out that help also takes additional work, by students who are already being required to invest more time and effort into their education than others. Especially for autistic students and those with some types of chronic illness, it may take more than usual effort to manage activities of daily living as well, and, far more often than with academic challenges, students are unwilling or unable to obtain institutional support for managing these types of need.[2] Attending higher education may be the first time in a student's life that they have been required to manage their own daily living needs independently, and making that (often unsupported) adjustment on top of meeting new academic requirements can be extremely overwhelming (Schwenk et al., 2014; Cage & Howes, 2020). In at least one study, students with ADHD report finding the already excessive demands on their time increased further by the need to hold a job while attending school, which is likely a factor in other categories as well (Melara, 2012). Students with chronic illnesses, on top

---

2   Simmeborn Fleischer, 2012; Cullen, 2013; Simmeborn Fleischer et al., 2013; Kreider et al., 2015; Toor et al., 2016; Anderson et al., 2017; LeGary, 2017; Hoffman et al., 2019.

of other time concerns, report needing to budget time into their schedules for the possibility of medical emergencies (Toller & Farrimond, 2021). Even if students may be able to achieve a balance between other factors and their academic lives, achieving and maintaining that balance is also a task that requires an investment of time and effort (Colclough, 2018; Spencer et al., 2018; Hoffman et al., 2019).

As a result of these outsized demands on their time and their physical and mental energy, many of these students are required to make adjustments and sacrifices in order to be successful academically, often to the significant detriment of their overall quality of life. Students across numerous studies and categories report having to forego social engagement, personal lives, and extracurricular activities simply to be able to keep up with the academic demands on their time.[3] Students in multiple studies describe taking even more extra time to work outside of classes and assignments, in order to try to keep from falling behind classmates, by reviewing lectures and other course materials, viewing instructional videos online, and other compensatory strategies (Pino & Mortari, 2014; MacCullagh et al., 2016). Although group work in classes can be very beneficial and desirable for students in several of these categories, a number of studies have observed that group projects can also be a major source of anxiety and discomfort for these students, because of the difficulties the extra demands on their time present in keeping pace with their fellow group members.[4] In a number of very real ways, the extra work that higher education demands from neurodivergent and invisibly disabled students not only increases their time pressures and stress, it prevents them from accessing the full college and university experience that is available to their nondisabled and neurotypical peers.

Institution and Curriculum

Another common experience reported by many disabled and neurodivergent students is that inequity begins for them from the very first step in the higher education process: choosing an institution to

---

3   Randolph, 2012; Couzens et al., 2015; Kreider et al., 2015; Lambert & Dryer, 2018; Ward & Webster, 2018; Gurbuz et al., 2019; Harn et al., 2019; Krumpelman & Hord, 2021.

4   Kreider et al., 2015; Pirttimaa et al., 2015; Stampoltzis et al., 2015; Giroux et al., 2020.

attend. Multiple studies have found that, depending on the nature of a student's specific needs, their choices of higher education institution may be driven by the relative availability of supports at a particular institution—or lack thereof at another.[5] This limitation was particularly frequently mentioned in studies of autistic students, although students with ADHD, TBI, and other considerations also reported making the same types of decision. Autistic students have specifically mentioned that they would advise similar students to choose an institution and discipline based on their needs as well as their interests, and also found other features of certain campuses to potentially influence their choices, such as small size or proximity to home (Anderson et al., 2020). Campus size and proximity to home were also common criteria for institutions chosen by students with other types of impairments (Flowers, 2012; Davis, 2019), and the layout of a campus, distances, and transportation issues have all been noted as significant potential barriers for students, particularly those with chronic illnesses (Redpath et al., 2013). While some of these elements may also be factors in college or university choice for nondisabled and neurotypical students, many neurodivergent and invisibly disabled students have to consider them as make-or-break factors in their ability to succeed in higher education, not merely as matters of preference. Moreover, having to calculate for institutions' widely varying levels of disability support and accessibility limits students' ability to choose their institutions based on other factors, like academic, social, and extracurricular interests.

Similar constraints apply to students' choices regarding academics. Across many studies, students report needing to reduce their own academic self-expectations in various ways to be able to advance through higher education, often at the cost of their interests and goals. Students may find they need to take a reduced courseload or only take one course at a time (Bush et al., 2011; Schindler & Kietz, 2013; Kain et al., 2019), change their course content, such as avoiding certain topics or intensive reading and writing requirements (Schindler & Kietz, 2013; Pirttimaa et al., 2015), or move to less demanding programs altogether.[6]

---

5   Flowers, 2012; Redpath et al., 2013; Accardo et al., 2019b; Davis, 2019; Anderson et al., 2020.

6   Childers & Hux, 2016; Anderson et al., 2018; Leopold et al., 2019; Anderson et al., 2020; Toller & Farrimond, 2021.

It should be stressed that, overall, these changes are not made due to their level of academic aptitude or diligence, but because of unavoidable factors inherent in the lives of the students in question. Autistic students in Anderson et al. (2018) who reported leaving their academic unit, for example, did so not because of a lack of affinity for the material, but explicitly because they were not consistently provided with the supports they needed to complete their work: they found that necessary accommodations were not available or simply not provided, they encountered negative experiences in trying to secure accommodations, or university staff failed to follow up to ensure their needs were actually met. As one student succinctly described their experience, "'[Got] my reasonable adjustment document on Friday of week 12 in a 13-week semester.'" (Anderson et al., 2018)

Disability Support Services

Studies have repeatedly found correlations between neurodivergent and invisibly disabled students' use of supports and accommodations and their academic success. Most commonly, access to accommodations has been found to be significantly correlated to persistence to graduation, based on quantitative data and systematic reviews of literature.[7] Additionally, across many interview studies, there is an overwhelming consensus among students themselves that accommodations are beneficial and support their academic success,[8] although care and appropriateness in implementation does affect the perceived helpfulness of the accommodations.[9]

As a result of these factors, it is concerning that, as quantitative studies and literature reviews have also shown, relatively few of these same students report accessing disability services and accommodations.

---

7   Pingry O'Neill et al., 2012; Koch et al., 2014; Kutscher & Tuckwiller, 2019; Clouder et al., 2020; Newman et al., 2021.

8   Erten, 2011; Heiney, 2011; Zafran et al., 2011; Flowers, 2012; Melara, 2012; Randolph, 2012; Mullins & Preyde, 2013; Rutherford, 2013; Ennals et al., 2015; Kreider et al., 2015; Cai & Richdale, 2016; Childers & Hux, 2016; Toor et al., 2016; Casement et al., 2017; Pitt & Soni, 2017; Sarrett, 2017; Berry, 2018; Kent et al., 2018; Lightfoot et al., 2018; Lizotte, 2018; Accardo et al., 2019b; Kain et al., 2019; Anderson et al., 2020; Thompson, 2021.

9   Hadley & Satterfield, 2013; Van Hees et al., 2015; Hoffman et al., 2019; Scheef et al., 2019.

Koch et al. (2014) found that less than 10% of students with psychiatric disabilities reported using accommodations, with 15% indicating that they needed extended time accommodations but had not received them. Newman and Madaus (2015) found that among students with any disability, while 95% had received at least one accommodation at the level of secondary schooling, only 23% had at the postsecondary level. McGregor et al. (2018) found that only around 33% of students with learning disabilities received accommodations. Barber and Williams (2021) found that less than half of women students with chronic illness surveyed had received accommodations, and in a literature review on autistic students, Krumpelman and Hord (2021) found that students frequently reported not using academic supports even when they were available. Furthermore, across multiple cases and categories, interview studies frequently found that neurodivergent and invisibly disabled students report not using disability services or accommodations, not having or seeking access to them, or even actively resisting the idea of using them.[10]

What stands in the way of students' receiving any accommodations, or all of the accommodations that they truly need? One of the most significant barriers across studies is that, for a variety of reasons, students are reluctant to seek out assistance, to disclose information about their needs, to identify themselves as disabled, or all of these. The issue of disclosure and help-seeking is a complex one that has been discussed broadly across the literature, and will be investigated in greater detail in the following sections. Many other barriers exist, however, that also prevent students from receiving the help they need from disability support services. One that also recurs frequently is lack of awareness: students either do not know that disability services are available, or do not know they would qualify.[11] Even when students are aware of accommodations, furthermore, the processes of qualifying for and obtaining them is often confusing and

---

10 Bush et al., 2011; Heiney, 2011; Melara, 2012; Tarallo, 2012; Downing, 2014; Ness et al., 2014; Kent, 2015; Sayman, 2015; Gottschall & Young, 2017; Anderson et al., 2018; Kent et al., 2018; Serry et al., 2018; Clouder et al., 2020; Barber & Williams, 2021; Maurer-Smolder et al., 2021.
11 Heiney, 2011; Demery et al., 2012; Cullen, 2013; Markoulakis & Kirsh, 2013; McEwan & Downie, 2013; Redpath et al., 2013; Rutherford, 2013; Kreider et al., 2015; Giroux et al., 2016; Goodman, 2017; Serry et al., 2018; Anderson et al., 2020; Owens, 2020; Maurer-Smolder et al., 2021; Pfeifer et al., 2021.

unfamiliar, which can discourage students from seeking supports from the outset, feeling that trying to muddle through unsupported would be easier than expending even more time and effort for uncertain returns.[12] Many students may use other campus supports rather than trying to navigate all the hurdles of obtaining accommodations, even when accommodations are demonstrably helpful (Richardson, 2021). Even if students do pursue disability services support, furthermore, many report difficulties with actually accessing accommodations,[13] including being told they do not qualify for services (Winberg et al., 2019) or having requests denied (J.B. Roberts et al., 2011). Complex bureaucratic procedures sometimes lead to significant delays, inconsistent application, or complete failures to provide accommodations even when they should theoretically be granted.[14]

In navigating these processes, some students also report negative experiences with disability services staff in general (Heiney, 2011; Hong, 2015; Lightfoot et al., 2018). Specifically, some found even these staff treated them with suspicion, disbelief, and other negative attitudes (Cai & Richdale, 2016; Spencer et al., 2018), or did not seem to have sufficient understanding of their individual conditions and needs.[15] These experiences are by no means universal, and many other students report more positive experiences and impressions of disability services staff (Lightfoot et al., 2018; Zeedyk et al., 2019). If students do have negative experiences with the same staff members who are most meant to understand and assist them, however, the impact on students' well-being and receipt of needed services has the potential to be devastating, as Heiney (2011) also notes. As will be discussed in later chapters, help-seeking can be particularly difficult and vulnerable for autistic students and those with psychiatric disabilities, and even one negative experience could dramatically decrease these students' likelihood of persisting until their needs are met (Demery et al., 2012). As Toller and Farrimond

---

12 J.B. Roberts et al., 2011; Mullins & Preyde, 2013; Strnadová et al., 2015; Childers & Hux, 2016; Sarrett, 2017; Berry, 2018; Lightfoot et al., 2018; Spencer et al., 2018; Winberg et al., 2019.

13 Habib et al., 2012; Koch et al., 2014; MacCullagh et al., 2016; Lightfoot et al., 2018; Maurer-Smolder et al., 2021.

14 Melara, 2012; Redpath et al., 2013; Stampoltzis et al., 2015; Bunch, 2016; Cai & Richdale, 2016; Sarrett, 2017; Anderson et al., 2018.

15 Lefler et al., 2016; Serry et al., 2018; Leopold et al., 2019; Barber & Williams, 2021.

(2021) observe, what students experience from disability services offices is sometimes a matter of luck in terms of which individual staff members work with them, and, when true, this is cause for serious concern about the equity of the process. As Hubbard (2011) notes, disability services offices are also likely to be underfunded or understaffed overall, to the detriment of the ability of even the best staff to meet students' needs.

Even when accommodations are successfully provided, meanwhile, in practice they may prove to be less helpful than students hope. Across many studies, students report receiving accommodations that were insufficient or poorly suited to their actual needs.[16] As Redpath et al. (2013) notes, sometimes the workarounds implemented to accommodate disabled students introduce additional complications that could have been avoided by simple flexibility in how to complete coursework, such as when a specialized testing environment is provided that creates additional barriers for a student, rather than allowing the student to be evaluated by other means than a test. The ways that accommodations are implemented can also place still more burdens on the students receiving them, such as requiring students to approach peers as potential note-takers rather than having note-takers selected for them (Hadley, 2017), or the frequent requirement that students present and negotiate their accommodation needs with faculty personally (Hoffman et al., 2019). Additionally, support outside of the academic curriculum may be difficult or impossible to obtain, either in students' perception or in fact.[17] In short, as a student in Erten (2011) observes with regard to accommodations: 'It is just so funny that it is perceived as privilege, when even it isn't equal' (p. 108). The many difficulties and shortcomings of accommodations alone should dispel the impression that these represent an 'unfair advantage' for disabled students—and yet that stigma persists, and creates another burden for students who do manage to obtain accommodations to bear.

---

16   Hubbard, 2011; Cullen, 2013; Stein, 2013; Gelbar et al., 2015; Hong, 2015; Cai & Richdale, 2016; Giroux et al., 2016; Lefler et al., 2016; Gottschall & Young, 2017; Lightfoot et al., 2018; Hoffman et al., 2019; Zeedyk et al., 2019; Barber & Williams, 2021; Maurer-Smolder et al., 2021; Thompson, 2021; Toller & Farrimond, 2021.

17   Cullen, 2013; Toor et al., 2016; Anderson & Butt, 2017; Clouder et al., 2020; Krumpelman & Hord, 2021.

Issues around Disclosure and Help-Seeking

Regardless of how much support they may need, students are often unwilling to disclose those needs to university administrators, faculty, and staff, even to obtain formal accommodations and other services. This is one of the most commonly recurring elements of the interviews and surveys examined. In some cases, a study will simply note the student's unwillingness or failure to obtain supports that would require acknowledgement of their disability or neurodivergence, with few details about reasoning provided, beyond that students were uncomfortable doing so.[18]

When there is information on why students choose not to disclose or seek help, however, certain reasons seem to recur over and over. By far the most common, across multiple studies and categories, is that students are afraid of being stigmatized if they disclose, either because they anticipate stigma, they have internalized stigma, or in many cases, because they have actually experienced stigma in the past.[19] In some cases, negative and stigmatizing experiences with peers have left lasting impressions on students, preventing or delaying them from seeking academic support (Winberg et al., 2019; Lett et al., 2020; Pfeifer et al., 2021). In other cases, faculty and staff interactions may have already borne out students' fear of stigma from authority figures in these roles. These concerns will be addressed in greater detail in Chapter 4. Some students hold the related fear that they will be disbelieved about their needs, often due to past experience (Bolourian et al., 2018; Spencer et al., 2018). The invisible nature of the categories presented here tends to contribute to students' unmet needs and to their being misunderstood.[20]

---

18   Demery et al., 2012; Anderson et al., 2018; Kent et al., 2018; Hoffman et al., 2019; Leopold et al., 2019; Owens, 2020; Barber & Williams, 2021; Krumpelman & Hord, 2021.

19   J.B. Roberts et al., 2011; Markoulakis & Kirsh, 2013; Mullins & Preyde, 2013; Redpath et al., 2013; Stein, 2013; Pino & Mortari, 2014; Hong, 2015; Pirttimaa, 2015; Timmerman & Mulvihill, 2015; Van Hees et al., 2015; Cai & Richdale, 2016; Lefler et al., 2016; Sokal & Desjardins, 2016; Toor et al., 2016; Anderson et al., 2017; Bolourian et al., 2018; Cox et al., 2017; Goodman, 2017; Lightfoot et al., 2018; Serry et al., 2018; Ward & Webster, 2018; Adams et al., 2019; Kain et al., 2019; Winberg et al., 2019; Clouder et al., 2020; Giroux et al., 2020; Grimes et al., 2020; James et al., 2020; Miller et al., 2020; Maurer-Smolder et al., 2021; Richardson, 2021.

20   Erten, 2011; Childers & Hux, 2016; Giroux et al., 2016; Anderson et al., 2018; Spencer et al., 2018; Zeedyk, 2019.

Another frequently recurring barrier to student disclosure and help-seeking is that students may feel that they are not needy or 'deserving' enough to merit support, and they may see (or feel that others see) accommodations as unfair advantages.[21] A number of studies demonstrate that students' fear of this perception is justified: Giroux et al. (2016) noted negative attitudes toward accommodations and even toward ill students when surveying faculty, and in multiple studies students recount lived experiences with peers who were resentful or skeptical of their accommodations and medications (particularly in the case of medication for ADHD) as perceived unfair advantages.[22] Even neurodivergent and disabled students themselves have clearly internalized these ideas in several studies, framing their own actual or potential accommodations as undeserved 'handouts,' which they may feel potentially compromise the worth of their education and degrees.[23] In one student's words:

> I have found it really difficult asking for help. I hate it. I guess it's just something psychological that I need to get past. I'll think, 'Why should I be advantaged?' 'No, no, no, you can't do that. It's wrong!' 'I'm cheating by taking this extension'. (Ward & Webster, 2018, p. 387)

Cameron & Billington (2017) particularly and usefully point out the neoliberal foundations of these ideas, rooted in a valorization of need-blind 'equality' over genuine equity in education—which many students have likely internalized from the pervasiveness of similar framings in their educational and social environments.

Similarly, another major reason that students do not disclose accommodation needs is their desire for independence, and the misplaced sense that institutional support would constitute undesirable dependence. In many interviews, students identified the desire to be independent or to succeed in college 'on their own' as a reason

---

21   J.B. Roberts et al., 2011; Markoulakis & Kirsh, 2013; Mullins & Preyde, 2013; Pino & Mortari, 2014; Couzens et al., 2015; Timmerman & Mulvihill, 2015; Spencer et al., 2018; Maurer-Smolder et al., 2021.

22   Young, 2012; Mullins & Preyde, 2013; Kreider et al., 2015; Gottschall & Young, 2017; Pfeifer et al., 2021.

23   Sayman, 2015; Childers & Hux, 2016; Lefler et al., 2016; Cameron & Billington, 2017; James et al., 2020.

for not seeking accommodations.[24] In some cases, students even described specifically wanting to complete their work without the use of supports,[25] or expressed that they equated the use of supports with dependence (MacCullagh et al., 2016; Sokal & Desjardins, 2016) or even 'cheating' (Sayman, 2015). Cameron and Billington (2017), along with Heiney (2011), again note the influence of neoliberal attitudes on this construction, in which students position individualism as paramount and themselves as solely responsible for their own success or failure in college. They also note that this construction therefore positions students who are less successful or have greater need as simply less hard-working or deserving, and fails to recognize the potential for solidarity between students who need support. It is not difficult to see how such ideas have infiltrated students' own self-understandings, either, when examining the framings sometimes employed even by the authors of these studies. Bush et al. (2011) and Hadley and Satterfield (2013), for example, seem particularly fixated on the need for students to be independent, and the concern that faculty and staff will 'over-accommodate' them—which is anything but borne out by the literature overall. Hadley (2017) even goes so far as to characterize a dyslexic and dysgraphic student's expressed desire for writing support—a very common academic support for disabled and nondisabled students alike—as 'dependence' (p. 24). With even some of their allies in academia configuring their support needs in these terms, it is not at all surprising that many students fear support would reflect on them poorly as independent learners.

A related barrier that prevents students from disclosing needs or seeking help is feeling embarrassment, shame, secrecy, or related emotions around their neurodivergence or disability (Hubbard, 2011; Lefler et al., 2016; Sokal & Desjardins, 2016). Likely due to heightened social stigma around psychiatric disabilities, this problem is mentioned especially frequently in the narratives of students with these conditions.[26] These students have been found to have a particular desire for privacy in academic services, including library services (Sokal & Desjardins,

---

24 Kirwan & Leather, 2011; Tarallo, 2012; Timmerman & Mulvihill, 2015; MacCullagh et al., 2016; Anderson et al., 2017; Bolourian et al., 2018; Serry et al., 2018; Anderson et al., 2020; Miller et al., 2020.
25 Melara, 2012; Ness et al., 2014; Kent et al., 2018; Adams et al., 2019.
26 Hubbard, 2011; Demery et al., 2012; Stein, 2013; Sokal & Desjardins, 2016.

2016; Pionke, 2017), and to be particularly unlikely to disclose their disabilities compared to students with other disabilities (Kent, 2015). Some students also note discomfort with seeking out disability services due to the possibility of hypervisibility or drawing unwanted attention to themselves (Mullins & Preyde, 2013), which may also in some cases be related to these concerns.

The need for self-advocacy that the support-seeking process demands is yet another significant barrier, often noted across the literature. A number of studies have found that self-advocacy skills and capacity are quite unevenly distributed across their student participants, with some students experiencing the need to self-advocate as a major struggle.[27] This is noted in several studies of autistic students, even when students are self-aware of the support that they need (Ward & Webster, 2018; Krumpelman & Hord, 2021). Lack of advocacy skills has even been found to be a major factor in non-completion for autistic students (Anderson et al., 2020). It is true that the capacity for self-advocacy is a positive and valuable skill, and many student narratives explicitly recognize this fact.[28] In a number of studies, furthermore, students found that their help-seeking and self-advocacy skills developed over time, as they increased their understanding of themselves and of what help was available.[29] Entering students seldom receive any explicit training in this skill, however, and as noted at the beginning of this chapter, a third of all disabled students leave college without return by their second year, meaning that for many, this growth never has time to occur. It is to their benefit when students do develop self-advocacy skills, but for these skills to be required in order to succeed in college at all is problematic to say the least, when they are so challenging for many and slow to develop. It is equally problematic to place the onus on disabled students to fight and persist just to access what they are legally entitled to, rather than to take responsibility for reducing the barriers that make self-advocacy so necessary.

---

27   Hubbard, 2011; Childers & Hux, 2016; Ward & Webster, 2018; Davis, 2019; Krumpelman & Hord, 2021.

28   Hubbard, 2011; Melara, 2012; Strnadova et al., 2015; Berry, 2018; Lightfoot et al., 2018; MacLeod et al., 2018; Accardo et al., 2019b; Davis, 2019.

29   Tarallo, 2012; Sayman, 2015; Childers & Hux, 2016; Lux, 2016; Berry, 2018; Bolourian et al., 2018; Davis, 2019; Harn et al., 2019.

Finally, even if students are willing to overcome all of these potential barriers, they often do not believe the supports or accommodations they would receive would be helpful.[30] As discussed above, this concern is in many cases justified, with the available institutional accommodations proving insufficient or ill-suited to the student's need. If students do not feel they can be confident that their experience with disability services will be sufficiently private or respectful of their needs, nor that it will result in support that will actually benefit them and address those needs, it is entirely reasonable that they may not choose to push past the many barriers and seek formal assistance. Instead, as reported in a number of studies, they are more likely to attempt to compensate on their own for their additional pressures, and self-disclose selectively only to specific course faculty or when their need is the greatest.[31]

Diagnosis and Categorization

Another complicating factor of seeking accommodations is that students are generally required to provide evidence of formal diagnosis with a disability in order to qualify. Obtaining a diagnosis from a medical professional, however, is not always a simple matter, especially when it comes to neurodivergence and invisible disabilities. Simply undergoing the medical processes required can be a significant barrier in terms of time, effort, and financial cost.[32] As noted by Winberg et al. (2019), the categories under discussion here also tend to present in highly diverse ways, meaning that a student's legitimate impairments may go misdiagnosed or undiagnosed because they vary from those of others with the same condition. Even when students are diagnosed, autistic students may be particularly likely to resist their diagnosis (Cox et al., 2021), while some students with ADHD and other neurodivergence classified as 'learning disabilities' may experience diagnosis as profoundly negative, even detrimental in itself (Lux et al., 2016)—although others may find it comes as a relief and an explanation for ongoing issues

---

30 Heiney, 2011; Tarallo, 2012; Anderson et al., 2017; Kent et al., 2018; Serry et al., 2018.

31 Melara, 2012; Schwenk et al., 2014; Barber & Williams, 2021; Turosak & Siwierka, 2021.

32 Cai & Richdale, 2016; Lightfoot et al., 2018; Anderson et al., 2020; Barber & Williams, 2021; Pfeifer et al., 2021; Toller & Farrimond, 2021.

(Young, 2012). In any case, the experience has a significant emotional as well as practical impact, and is frequently reported as a major hurdle to pass before receiving support.

Compounding this challenge is the fact that students may or may not have received a diagnosis prior to college at all, and may not even be aware that there is anything to diagnose. Late diagnosis is common in the categories under discussion here, relative to other types of disability.[33] In Lizotte (2018) and Cage and Howes (2020), multiple student participants had not even been diagnosed until after finishing college. Students with psychiatric disabilities, in particular, have been found to be far less likely than those with other types of disabilities to be diagnosed during primary or secondary education, leading to lack of supports, lack of knowledge of their own needs, and sometimes not even realizing that they have unique needs that could be met (Hubbard, 2011; McEwan & Downie, 2013; Stein, 2013). Diagnosis can also be particularly delayed for autistic women, due to stereotypical association of autistic traits with men, and gendered differences in how autism tends to manifest (Cage & Howes, 2020; Krumpelman & Hord, 2021). This not only impacts students in higher education, but is also likely to have impacted their previous schooling experiences, affecting their level of academic performance, their resulting preparation for college, and even their psychological well-being. Earlier diagnosis has been linked to more positive self-acceptance and academic success (Pitt & Soni, 2017; Cipolla, 2018; Lightfoot et al., 2018) and greater readiness for managing invisible physical illness (Schwenk et al., 2014). Some autistic students specifically report that experiencing late diagnosis was a barrier to their success (Accardo et al., 2019b). Furthermore, students who were not diagnosed prior to reaching higher education consequently did not have documentation or allotted accommodations in their secondary schooling, meaning they did not enter college with plans or expectations for similar supports, or foreknowledge that they might need to seek out disability services (Hubbard, 2011; Flowers, 2012; Sarrett, 2017). Some students report that these disadvantages had made them feel they were not able to fully access and benefit from their primary and secondary education (Hubbard, 2011), and some had experienced resulting lack of self-understanding and low self-esteem, or had even been told they

---

33   Hubbard, 2011; Young, 2012; Doikou-Avlidou, 2015; Sarrett, 2017.

were 'stupid' rather than working at a genuine disadvantage (Hubbard, 2011; Sarrett, 2017). While higher education faculty and staff cannot retroactively remedy these past experiences, they should certainly take them into consideration as factors in the support these students may need, and the challenges they may face.

Disability Identity

Related to the issue of diagnosis is the issue of disability identity, and how it affects students' support-seeking, self-advocacy, and overall well-being. In student narratives in a number of studies, the idea of using accommodations was in tension with students' self-conceptions as either not disabled at all, or not having significant need compared to others with disabilities.[34] In fact, students in several studies specifically report not seeking out disability services because they did not consider themselves to be disabled (Downing, 2014; Timmerman & Mulvihill, 2015; Goodman, 2017). Students in the categories discussed here are, across multiple studies, frequently reluctant to identify themselves as disabled, or are resistant to that categorization.[35] This is an unfortunate fact in many respects, because, in numerous studies, positive disability identity has been linked to greater academic success, and increased likelihood of accessing academic supports and developing effective coping strategies (Erten, 2011; Kreider et al., 2015; Clouder et al., 2020). Stronger disability identity has also been cited as mitigating negative impacts on academic self-esteem and self-confidence that students experience as a result of their learning difficulties (Brandt & McIntyre, 2016).

Many neurodivergent and invisibly disabled students, however, do not feel able to claim the disability identity that would help support them in these ways. Lower disability identity and more ambivalence around one's diagnosis are especially frequently reported across studies of autistic students,[36] and of those with psychiatric disabilities (Kent,

---

34 Mullins & Preyde, 2013; Timmerman & Mulvihill, 2015; Cox et al., 2017; Spencer et al., 2018.

35 Heiney, 2011; Hubbard, 2011; Melara, 2012; Kreider et al., 2015; Sayman, 2015; Goodman, 2017; Clouder et al., 2020; James et al., 2020; Cox et al., 2021.

36 Simmeborn Fleischer, 2012; Downing, 2014; Sayman, 2015; MacLeod et al., 2018; Cox et al., 2021.

2015; Sayman, 2015; Goodman, 2017). It is worth noting, however, that as with self-advocacy skills, for many students disability identity tends to develop over time. During their time in college, students across a number of studies found that they gradually embraced a disability identity over time, integrating an increasing understanding of their own characteristics and needs into their sense of self.[37] Requiring students to self-report disabilities to receive institutional support, however, means that students' success may directly depend on their self-identification as disabled—which renders even a temporary resistance to this identity problematic for students, especially in the earlier, foundational years of higher education.

As Spencer et al. (2018) note, students all too often seem to find themselves caught between not wanting to identify as ill or disabled, but feeling compelled to do so nonetheless in order to be believed by faculty and staff, and to receive the supports that they need. The status of 'healthy' is valorized and prioritized socially in general, and chronically ill students internalize those values, making them seek to construct their own identity as 'healthy' and the traits that disable them as incidental. This makes the seeking of supports not only a significant practical challenge, but a potential identity crisis as well. It also seems apparent, given other components of the narratives of neurodivergent and invisibly disabled students, that a great deal of their resistance to a disability identity is due to the justified fear of the stigma and discrimination faced by people with that identity.

Whether a student identifies as disabled or not is a personal and individual matter, but it is of serious concern if students eschew this identity primarily because of how they may be treated because of it, and to their cost. It is also of note that when disability is stigmatized in higher education, and as a result students are unwilling to identify as disabled to seek support, this directly serves the interests of institutions reluctant to invest the time and effort needed to improve services for disabled students. I do not mean to suggest that university faculty and staff, when they do so, cause students to feel judged, ashamed, and belittled for disclosing disabilities in order to intentionally prevent those students from seeking disability support services from the university.

---

37   (Hubbard, 2011; Zafran et al., 2011; Ennals et al., 2015; Lux, 2016; Bolourian et al., 2018; Cage & Howes, 2020.

I do believe, however, that if university systems are set up to provide these types of services only reluctantly, this cannot help but influence the attitudes and behavior of many university employees.

Summary and Conclusions

While the campus environment may not hinder invisibly disabled and neurodivergent students as obviously as it can other disabled students, such as those who use mobility devices or have impairments of perception, their access to higher education is nevertheless definitively more limited and more difficult than that of nondisabled and neurotypical students. Students across all categories under discussion here experience substantially outsized demands on their time and energy in higher education, often to the point of having to limit or entirely forego non-academic activities. Their choices of course content, course modality, department and program, and even institution are likely to be limited artificially by which choice they feel will be able to meet their needs, rather than being freely made based on their academic interests and personal preferences. Furthermore, while many neurodivergent and invisibly disabled students may encounter barriers in the process of seeking accommodations, many others opt not to identify themselves or pursue support at all. This is not an irrational decision on the part of students: it is informed by their experiences of how they may be treated if they disclose their needs, and by prevailing attitudes about who is and is not 'deserving' of support, how support is equated to dependence, and how needing certain types of support is perceived as shameful. Even if they should decide to conquer all of these concerns, they are forced to advocate for themselves aggressively and persistently to receive support, which many are unequipped to do. It is also often unclear to them what support is available and how it would be helpful, causing them to lack confidence that this substantial effort would be worthwhile. Compounding these difficulties are the facts that invisibly disabled and neurodivergent students may not have received a diagnosis at all prior to college, or even during college, and may not be aware of what their needs are, let alone able to provide evidence of diagnosis to qualify for accommodations. Even if they have been diagnosed, they may feel significant ambivalence toward or even resist the diagnosis, and in many cases may not identify as disabled at all, making them unlikely to seek out supports that are identified as being for students with disabilities. The ability of students to manage all of these factors does appear to increase over time, but when more than one-third of students with disabilities permanently withdraw from college within their first two years, it is clear that many students are not able to persist long enough under these conditions for that growth to occur.

It is a choice to frame higher education this way. It is a choice to offer a singular educational experience, dictated by the judgment of faculty and staff, the requirements of which students must either meet as they are and unaided, or by requesting workarounds that will help them overcome the parts of the standard mold they find most insurmountable—and then require them to offer justification and proof of why they need and deserve even that much flexibility. Like students' choice to avoid disclosing their needs and asking for help, it is not an irrational choice, and there are practical, philosophical, and historical reasons for these procedures to be in place. Like many students' choices described here, though, it is also not a choice that results in equitable educational experiences. The neurodivergent and invisibly disabled students who are able to succeed in this environment are not definitionally those who are most academically capable, but those who are most fortunate. Students can succeed if, by chance, they happen to be able to persist through bureaucratic systems, identify and make the case for their own needs, brave the social stigma around those needs, and access medical treatment and diagnosis—or else exert all of the extra time and effort required to compensate for those needs without any formal support at all. Those unable to do either of these things will not even have the opportunity to prove their capability for academic work and learning. They will fail at the format.

This is not the only way that supporting disabled students in higher education could work. Pursuing a more equitable environment for neurodivergent and invisibly disabled students can begin with reframing how support is made available, from 'students who need it can get help on request' to proactively seeking on the university side to eliminate barriers, increase flexibility, and make supports independently available for all students, regardless of their needs or how they self-identify.

These are the principles behind Universal Design, whether in the form of Universal Design for Learning (UDL) or other forms of design. The more an institution's culture is able to shift in this direction, the less any given student's self-advocacy skills, diagnosis, or disability identity will matter to their ability to be successful in higher education. It is not a simple matter to shift the design of systems and policies this way, but it is a shift from which every part of the institution can benefit—including, as will be discussed next, the classroom environment itself.

4. Curriculum and Classroom

Academic courses are the center of college and university life, around which many other elements are organized. Progressing through course work is ostensibly the main purpose of students' enrollment, regardless of what larger goals that work may serve. As discussed in Chapter 3, course work places major demands on the time and effort of neurodivergent and invisibly disabled students, often to the exclusion of social and other life activities. The factors that support and inhibit students' success in their courses, therefore, are some of the most important in higher education overall. Furthermore, in student accounts of their experiences in higher education, a large number of the issues and needs they most commonly note have to do with faculty relations, study, and other aspects of their course-based academic work.

In this chapter, the focus will be on aspects of the curriculum and classroom, particularly those that neurodivergent students and those with invisible disabilities most commonly report finding valuable or difficult to manage. There is a wide array of factors to consider, but most fall roughly into three categories:

1. The attitudes, behavior, and interventions of faculty;
2. Students' commonly reported academic strengths and weaknesses; and
3. Elements of course design that bear on students' needs.

While this chapter by no means exhaustively addresses accessibility concerns in course design, the issues highlighted are those that seem to recur the most frequently in student narratives of their experiences.

    https://doi.org/10.11647/OBP.0420.04

Faculty Attitudes and Support

Experiences with faculty dominate students' narratives of their higher education experiences, not surprisingly. Faculty play a critical role in students' success in college, and how a given faculty member relates to students can be vital in how a student experiences one course, or even an entire subject. It is concerning, therefore, that so many students' narratives describe profoundly negative incidents with course faculty. Students frequently report encountering faculty members who seem to have little awareness of disabilities in general, invisible disabilities in particular, or the student's specific condition or neurodivergence.[1] Negative attitudes held by faculty toward students with disabilities are also frequently reported, whether these were perceived by students or otherwise.[2] For example, Giroux et al. (2016) found that past surveys had identified patterns of negative attitudes toward students with chronic illnesses by faculty members. Students also frequently report experiences with faculty members who were reluctant to comply with their requests for accommodations, refused to provide the supports to which students were legally entitled, would not provide any flexibility with format and structural elements of course assignments, or combinations of these.[3] In some cases, faculty cited 'unfairness' to other students as a reason for the refusal, indicating a lack of understanding of the purpose and nature of accommodations (Pino & Mortari, 2014; Kreider et al., 2015; Giroux et al., 2016). Faculty are also frequently experienced as unresponsive and unsupportive when students make accommodation requests, sometimes simply because of overwork or lack of availability.[4] A number of studies also found these types of issues

---

1   Erten, 2011; Randolph, 2012; Mullins & Preyde, 2013; Redpath et al., 2013; Heindel, 2014; Stampoltzis, 2015; Sarrett, 2017; Winberg et al., 2019; Accardo et al., 2019b; Clouder et al., 2020; Turosak & Siwierka, 2021.

2   Erten, 2011; Gallo et al., 2014; Pino & Mortari, 2014; Hong, 2015; Pirttimaa, 2015; Stampoltzis, 2015; Turosak & Siwierka, 2021.

3   Hubbard, 2011; J.B. Roberts et al., 2011; Randolph, 2012; Mullins & Preyde, 2013; Redpath et al., 2013; Catalano, 2014; Pino & Mortari, 2014; Pirttimaa, 2015; Stampoltzis, 2015; Strnadova et al., 2015; Sokal & Desjardins, 2016; Lizotte, 2018; Winberg et al., 2019; Accardo et al., 2019b; Pfeifer et al., 2021.

4   Hadley & Satterfield, 2013; Rutherford, 2013; Gallo et al., 2014; Pino & Mortari, 2014; Sokal & Desjardins, 2016; White et al., 2016; Lightfoot et al., 2018; Accardo et al., 2019b; Clouder et al., 2020; Cox et al., 2021; Pfeifer et al., 2021.

to be a significant factor in dealing with academic support staff, such as advisors (Markoulakis & Kirsh, 2013; Hong, 2015; Woof, 2021).

In many cases, moreover, a faculty member who is unsupportive or who hesitates to implement accommodations may be exhibiting some of the least negative behavior that students encounter. Student narratives across many studies also describe experiences of disclosing a disability or neurodivergence to faculty or staff, and receiving a response that was stigmatizing, discriminatory, or even abusive.[5] A student in Houman and Stapley (2013), for example, describes an experience where a faculty member was vocally critical during class of the student's appearance of illness and exhaustion, even when the student had previously disclosed a chronic health condition with fatigue as a symptom.

A nonverbal autistic student in Ashby and Causton-Theoharis (2012) who uses facilitated communication described a particularly egregious incident:

> While he was not the only one to question her typing, this professor actually included the practice of facilitated communication as an example of a "bizarre belief." When I asked her to explain how she knew her faculty did not believe in her typing she responded, "It was not hard to tell. One teacher included it in the curriculum. FC as bizarre." (p. 274)

Especially for students with psychiatric disabilities, encounters with teaching faculty in some cases can be so demeaning, humiliating, and antagonistic that they trigger psychiatric symptoms and avoidance of academic coursework (Hubbard, 2011; Hong, 2015; Giroux et al., 2020).

The many demoralizing experiences that students describe are particularly frustrating because their positive experiences have an equally dramatic impact. When faculty and staff are supportive and compassionate, those experiences are transformatively valuable for students, just as negative experiences can be debilitating.[6] Students in

---

5   Heiney, 2011; Ashby & Causton-Theoharis, 2012; Habib et al., 2012; Wilson, 2012; Markoulakis & Kirsh, 2013; Gallo et al., 2014; Doikou-Avlidou, 2015; Kreider et al., 2015; Pirttimaa, 2015; Timmerman & Mulvihill, 2015; Brandt & McIntyre, 2016; Anderson et al., 2018; Bolourian et al., 2018; Hoffman et al., 2019; Kain et al., 2019; Zeedyk, 2019; Clouder et al., 2020; Giroux et al., 2020; Pfeifer et al., 2021; Thompson, 2021; Turosak & Siwierka, 2021.

6   Heiney, 2011; Randolph, 2012; Wilson, 2012; Rutherford, 2013; Schindler & Kietz, 2013; Gelbar et al., 2014; Pino & Mortari, 2014; Strnadova et al., 2015; Childers & Hux, 2016; Giroux et al., 2016; LeGary, 2017; Smith, 2017; Cipolla, 2018; Colclough, 2018; Lightfoot et al., 2018; Serry et al., 2018; Ward & Webster, 2018; Kain et al.,

some studies have cited supportive faculty as a major factor in their academic success (Ward & Webster, 2018; Kutscher & Tuckwiller, 2019). Students in Smith (2017) mention supportive faculty as a valued source of emotional support, as well as academic, and students in Colclough (2018) make particular note of the beneficial effects of positive relationships with faculty. Overwhelmingly, faculty support is consistently listed as one of the most valued supports for students, while unsupportive and obstructive faculty are consistently listed as one of the most significant barriers. It is not an exaggeration to say that how faculty and staff respond to students can make or break those students' experiences of a course, a subject, or university as a whole. The fact that so many miss this chance to directly support student success is therefore extremely disappointing.

Many of these issues are exacerbated by the common requirement in higher education that students with accommodations present these to faculty personally for negotiation, without the buffer of disability services staff. There are certainly reasons that institutions have made the choice to implement this requirement, and not all of them stem from underfunded, understaffed, and otherwise under-resourced disability services offices. In theory, engaging faculty in these conversations could help students to build important skills in self-advocacy, as well as a greater understanding of their own needs through having to repeatedly articulate them. In practice, however, many factors confound the good intentions behind making students their own advocates, as has been noted in the previous chapter. For many students, particularly those who are neurodivergent or invisibly disabled in the ways addressed here, these interactions represent extremely anxiety-producing communication challenges (Rutherford, 2013; Pfeifer et al., 2021), especially for autistic students (Cai & Richdale, 2016). As noted in Kreider et al. (2015), many students feel that the need to self-disclose to faculty constitutes requiring them to disclose private medical information to faculty in order to access their allotted supports. This perception can be exacerbated by faculty and staff who are invasive and inappropriate in follow-up questioning (Heindel, 2014; Zeedyk, 2019), or who are inattentive to confidentiality in discussing accommodations with students, such as mentioning their

---

2019; Kutscher & Tuckwiller, 2019; Lipka et al., 2019; Anderson et al., 2020; Giroux et al., 2020; Owens, 2020; Cox et al., 2021; Pfeifer et al., 2021.

conditions or support needs in front of classmates without permission (Melara, 2012; Pfeifer et al., 2021). Put together, all of these concerns make approaching faculty about course accommodations a major emotional barrier, one that students tend to avoid as much as possible, choosing instead to muddle through without even the accommodations to which they are formally entitled (Melara, 2012; Kreider et al., 2015; Stampoltzis, 2015). Negative experiences with faculty regarding their support needs also tend to make neurodivergent and invisibly disabled students less likely to approach those faculty for help outside of class, deterring them from types of academic support that would normally be available to any student (Gallo et al., 2014).

Beyond these most significant issues around faculty attitudes and behavior, there are also more minor logistical improvements faculty could make to their course management to increase support. For example, students also frequently mention the value they place on faculty feedback. A number of students agree that feedback from an instructor on their academic work is extremely important to them, but that the feedback they do receive is frequently insufficient to be helpful (LeGary, 2017; Smith, 2017; Jansen et al., 2018). Another area where more instructor intervention would be beneficial is in the implementation of group projects. Group work can be highly beneficial for students with all types of learning needs, as students themselves recognize (if sometimes reluctantly) in their narratives (Tarallo, 2012; Stampoltzis, 2015; Harn et al., 2019). In some cases, it may even serve as a support in itself: for example, students with ADHD in Flowers (2012) indicated that they were able to be most successful in classes where they could engage in group work, as opposed to those in a lecture format. As noted in Chapter 3, however, the excessive and frequently unpredictable time demands on neurodivergent students and those with invisible disabilities can make it difficult to keep pace with a group of their peers, which may lead to misunderstandings, tensions, and resentment if not properly managed (Kreider et al., 2015; Pirttimaa, 2015; Stampoltzis, 2015). Autistic students and those with psychiatric disabilities are also more likely to have difficulty with the social components of group projects, making these experiences more difficult and uncomfortable to navigate without assistance.[7] While this does not mean that group work ought to be eliminated entirely, particularly given its positive effects, it does mean that it needs to be implemented with great care and thoughtfulness to mitigate potential negative impacts for the more vulnerable members of the class. Indeed, as suggested by Cullen (2013) and demonstrated in Gelbar et al. (2014), the class may be best served by faculty support and even direct intervention in project groups, to ensure their smooth functioning.

Academic Strengths and Weaknesses

Information Processing Challenges

Absorbing, interpreting, and communicating information effectively is ascribed critical importance in higher education, which makes it a significant disadvantage that students in several categories particularly struggle with these tasks. Information processing issues are a common theme across student narratives, and are due to technical challenges of their impairments, rather than any lack of aptitude or effort. Dyslexic students, as one might assume, mostly report struggles with heavy reading and writing requirements in higher education courses, and, even with various types of support, reading and writing are still more time-consuming and cumbersome for them than for other students.[8] This problem is exacerbated by how higher education assignments often unthinkingly default to the written word as a means of disseminating and evaluating learning, even when reading and writing skills are not the core content to be learned, and other delivery modes might be just as effective (Mullins & Preyde, 2013). For example, group work can be a very helpful learning practice for these students (Clouder et al., 2020), and options to take examinations orally can be helpful as well, although in some cases this depends on the individual student (Stampoltzis, 2015; Serry et al., 2018).

---

7   Tarallo, 2012; Cullen, 2013; Rutherford, 2013; Knott & Taylor, 2014; Kent, 2015; Cai & Richdale, 2016; Toor et al., 2016; Anderson et al., 2017; Gurbuz et al., 2019; Harn et al., 2019.

8   Hadley & Satterfield, 2013; Pino & Mortari, 2014; MacCullagh et al., 2016; Hadley, 2017; Maurer-Smolder et al., 2021; Richardson, 2021.

Autistic students, meanwhile, report a more varied set of challenges with taking in information. Some autistic students report auditory processing issues,[9] while others struggle with navigating neurotypical-centric structures of information. Some of the challenges described in this area include difficulty interpreting information that is not organized according to an explicit structure (Jansen et al., 2018), and difficulty determining the relative importance and context of information (Jansen et al., 2018; Clouder et al., 2020). Similarly, autistic students may tend to take in more information less discriminatingly than their neurotypical counterparts, struggling more to filter out irrelevant information in class materials and academic environments (Everhart & Escobar, 2018). They may also find that they think and understand in particularly linear and literal ways that are sometimes incompatible with their academic requirements (Cox et al., 2021).

Students with ADHD also report a similar variety of issues with absorbing and expressing information. Participants in several studies report needing extra time to process information in general (Hubbard, 2011; Catalano, 2014; James et al., 2020), as well as difficulties and discomfort with expressing their thoughts in writing (Hubbard, 2011; Catalano, 2014). Some students with ADHD also report issues with communication in general (Melara, 2012; Wright, 2011), although in other cases their self-assessments are more variable (Hubbard, 2011). In still other cases, furthermore, students with ADHD actually find that their tendency to ruminate on abstract concepts at length can be to their academic benefit, especially in STEM fields—although this still presumes that they actually have time for this additional processing, which is not always the case (James et al., 2020).

Information processing issues are also common among students with traumatic brain injuries (TBI). Even across a variety of different personal backgrounds and types of brain injuries, students with TBI frequently report taking longer to think and process information than average (Bush et al., 2011; Childers & Hux, 2016; Owens, 2020), as well as struggling to process oral and visual information (Gotschall & Young, 2017; Owens, 2020). Some also experience difficulties with communication, whether these are noted by the students themselves or

---

9   Van Hees et al., 2015; Jansen et al., 2018; Anderson et al., 2020; Clouder et al., 2020.

by others (Bush et al., 2011; Owens, 2020). Interviews with a group of specifically female students with TBI also revealed post-injury difficulty with analyzing information, and with expressing themselves in writing (Gottschall & Young, 2017). All of these challenges, like those reported by students in other categories, present significant additional barriers to completing academic work.

Note-taking, for example, represents one specific academic task that is made significantly more difficult by these issues. Taking notes in class is a skill dyslexic students report finding especially difficult, and where accommodations are needed.[10] Not all students who need these supports receive them, however, and even when they are available, their perceived helpfulness may be questionable (Serry et al., 2018). Some students also specifically mention access to video or audio lecture recordings as beneficial in working around note-taking challenges (Pino & Mortari, 2014; Stampoltzis, 2015; Maurer-Smolder et al., 2021). Taking notes on course readings is challenging as well, and some students find they need to digitize print readings, or print digital readings, in order to take notes and manipulate these materials in the ways that they need (MacCullagh et al., 2016). A number of autistic students also report struggling with note-taking and needing support (Anderson et al., 2017; Accardo et al., 2019a; Accardo et al., 2019b), but how these services are delivered can affect their helpfulness (Accardo et al., 2019a).

Another common and related area of difficulty is with working memory, particularly in students with dyslexia, ADHD, or both concurrently. ADHD and dyslexia overlap significantly in how memory affects academic performance, and not least because it is fairly common for a student to be diagnosed with both. Students report specific difficulties with storage and recall of information (Cameron, 2016), as well as focus and motivation issues, especially in long classes or when completing long readings.[11] Many students also report using strategies to employ visual, aural, and other sensory forms of memory in order to compensate for these difficulties,[12] while others express a desire to learn these types of strategies (Serry et al., 2018). Numerous students

---

10   Olofsson et al., 2012; Pino & Mortari, 2014; Stampoltzis, 2015; MacCullagh et al., 2016; Smith, 2017; Clouder et al., 2020; Maurer-Smolder et al., 2021.

11   Wennås Brante, 2013; MacCullagh et al., 2016; Serry et al., 2018; Richardson, 2021.

12   Wilson, 2012; Pirttimaa, 2015; Cipolla, 2018; Richardson, 2021.

also mention the value of having the technological ability to adjust the speed at which information is presented, such as being able to slow down or pause a lecture recording, to help with memory issues (Pino & Mortari, 2014; MacCullagh et al., 2016; Maurer-Smolder et al., 2021). Similarly, students also report difficulties with organization in study and classwork, and using visual, aural, kinetic, and practical strategies to compensate, such as color-coding, flow-charting, and technological means of staying organized.[13] These difficulties are significant enough, however, that dyslexic students also report difficulty navigating other systems of organization on campus, such as academic libraries (Redpath et al., 2013; Stampoltzis, 2015). More often than dyslexic students, meanwhile, students with ADHD describe difficulties with executive function, focus, and memory. These include initiating work and staying on task, maintaining focus, and staying organized.[14] This seems to be especially true in online courses (J.B. Roberts et al., 2011). Some students also describe issues with short-term memory and forgetfulness, which may be related to distractibility (Hubbard, 2011; Melara, 2012; Schaffer, 2013).

Cycling, Variable, and Invisible Conditions

Many of the impairments under discussion here are not consistent over time in how much they impact students' lives. A chronically ill student may have a few weeks of significantly improved health and then a few of entirely disabling pain and fatigue, for example, or a student with ADHD may find their symptoms and needs have shifted significantly with maturation from what they were in secondary schooling, or a student with psychiatric disabilities may be well one day and unable to get out of bed the next. Students across multiple categories describe experiencing these variable patterns, although they are most commonly reported by those with psychiatric disabilities and chronic illness.[15] As one chronically ill student described it:

---

13 Pino & Mortari, 2014; Stampoltzis, 2015; Cameron & Greenland, 2021; Maurer-Smolder et al., 2021.

14 Hubbard, 2011; Roberts, 2011; Wright, S.A., 2011; Melara, 2012; Schaffer, 2013; Lefler et al., 2016; Kwon et al., 2018; James et al., 2020.

15 Mullins & Preyde, 2013; Ennals et al., 2015; Giroux et al., 2020; Toller & Farrimond, 2021; Turosak & Siwierka, 2021.

> Even if I plan and break everything down and stuff, I can just have a random week out of nowhere I can't do any work and I can't control that [...] it can be quite difficult emotionally, like not having that control and not being able to do anything about it. (Toller & Farrimond, 2021, under section header "The chronically ill body: a barrier to studying").

This can be especially problematic because these experiences are mismatched with nondisabled people's common understandings of disability, which tend to view impairment as something that either exists or does not, and is fixed and unchangeable. Even more obvious types of impairment, like those of mobility or vision and hearing, are often more complex than this construction allows, and neurodivergent and invisibly disabled people tend to experience even more unpredictability in their conditions than others. This can make it difficult to plan and commit to an entire semester's worth of uninterrupted work, and forces students into often taxing and suboptimal study patterns to compensate. For example, students may have to adjust their coping and study strategies multiple times a semester to manage the cycling of their symptoms, or work in a 'boom and bust' pattern of intense academic work during periods of lighter symptoms, followed by periods of decline and incapacity afterward—which may be partly triggered by the previous exhaustion and overwork (Toller & Farrimond, 2021). The unpredictability of these conditions may also lead to conflict with faculty, staff, and peers who do not understand these inconsistencies, and may even suspect or accuse students of deliberately underperforming or malingering during their most difficult periods (Toller & Farrimond, 2021).

On a related note, the invisibility of these conditions itself can create problems for students, many of which have been noted in their narratives. Most commonly, students describe encountering added barriers to obtaining the accommodations and other support they need for their conditions, because those conditions are either overlooked or outright challenged and disbelieved.[16] Depending on the institutional climate, battle fatigue from having to repeatedly defend the validity of an invisible condition may become a further drain on students' already limited time and energy (Giroux et al., 2016), or students' needs may simply go unmet if they do not have the will or capacity to keep fighting

---

16 Childers & Hux, 2016; Giroux et al., 2016; Anderson et al., 2018; Spencer et al., 2018; Zeedyk, 2019.

(Anderson et al., 2018). Some students also find that their peers are judgmental and unsympathetic about their conditions, due to not understanding the hardships invisible disabilities and neurodivergence can create (Erten, 2011). As much as students may feel the need to mask their symptoms and behavior, that mask can prevent them from obtaining much-needed support at the same time that it protects them from vulnerability.

Another related challenge is a spiral effect that is sometimes experienced by autistic and psychiatrically disabled students at times when they are struggling. It is a common pattern with these students that academic stress and falling behind with studies can worsen problematic symptoms and impairments, and vice versa; this vicious cycle can eventually lead students into complete crisis academically and personally if not interrupted.[17] Interruption is made far more difficult, however, by how autistic students frequently report a tendency to withdraw from others during periods of greater stress and difficulty, rather than reaching out for help.[18] As Ward and Webster (2018) incisively put it regarding autistic student study participants, when they 'were most in need of help, they were the least likely to request it' (p. 387), most often due to fear of stigma and guilt over 'bothering' university staff with difficulties they felt they should be able to self-manage. When autistic students are struggling, they may face even greater difficulty in resolving the issues without proactive external support, and this may be true of students in other categories as well.

Individual Strategies and Motivations

While students' self-described strengths tend to vary by category just as their weaknesses do, there are some notable recurring patterns across each. For one, when students understand their own individual needs, academic or otherwise, and develop personally tailored strategies to manage them, they report significant positive impacts. This seems to be

---

17 Hubbard, 2011; Markoulakis & Kirsh, 2013; Ennals et al., 2015; Anderson & Butt, 2017; LeGary, 2017; Bolourian et al., 2018; Ward & Webster, 2018; Anderson et al., 2020; Turosak & Siwierka, 2021.

18 Bolourian et al., 2018; Ward & Webster, 2018; Winberg et al., 2019; Clouder et al., 2020; Cox et al., 2021.

most reported in studies of students with ADHD[19] and autistic students,[20] but also in those of students with TBI (Ness et al., 2014; Davis, 2019; Owens, 2020), with dyslexia (Doikou-Avlidou, 2015; Stampoltzis, 2015; Thompson, 2021), and with psychiatric disabilities (Ennals et al., 2015; Kain et al., 2019; Turosak & Siwierka, 2021), as well as chronically ill students (Barber & Williams, 2021; Toller & Farrimond, 2021). An early sense of disability identity and strong self-awareness appears to support the development of these types of strategies (Erten, 2011). Students also need to have the time and space to develop strategies, along with other types of academic skills (Flowers, 2012). It is worth noting, as well, that sometimes no self-management strategy is sufficient to overcome a particularly severe challenge, impairment, or disabling environment (Heiney, 2011).

Similarly, while lack of academic motivation is reported as a challenge for students in some categories, particularly autistic and psychiatrically disabled students (Markoulakis & Kirsh, 2013; Schindler & Kietz, 2013; Cage & Howes, 2020), many students report developing successful self-motivation strategies to overcome this. For autistic students, lack of motivation has been found to be mitigated by their interest in particular career aspirations (Tarallo, 2012), or by setting specific goals for themselves (Accardo et al., 2019b). Veteran students with psychiatric disabilities also seem to be at an advantage over others in terms of managing low motivation, as military training is also cited as a mitigating factor (Ness et al., 2014). These students and others, however, may also benefit from seeking out additional sources of motivation to support them through their academic work. This is particularly true because motivation is frequently cited across studies as a significant factor in student success, especially for these students in particular (Zafran et al., 2011; Anderson et al., 2020).

Other students across various categories and studies describe a variety of motivating factors that aid in their success. One frequently cited motivator is the very practical one of the student's career and financial aspirations. Students recognize that college is a societal expectation for many career paths, and thus their determination to

---

19   Heiney, 2011; Kirwan & Leather, 2011; Melara, 2012; Schaffer, 2013; Lux et al., 2016; Lightfoot et al., 2018; James et al., 2020.

20   Toor et al., 2016; Ward & Webster, 2018; Accardo et al., 2019b; Anderson et al., 2020.

complete a degree stems from a clear view of its utility for the future.[21] Another common motivator is a positive attitude toward, and personal pride or pleasure in, educational achievement (Drake, 2014; Lambert & Dryer, 2018; Lightfoot et al., 2018); even when students do not cite this as a motivating factor specifically; there is also a general sense across the majority of studies that students generally regard higher education as a worthy, positive pursuit in itself, and one in which they would like to be successful. In particular, some students want to be successful in higher education in order to make family proud (Schaffer, 2013), or to honor the support they have received from friends and family (Bunch, 2016). Education can also be a positive and enjoyable part of life for students with psychiatric disabilities, by being a source of structure and meaning-making (Ennals et al., 2015), or a way of forming social connections (Ness et al., 2014). Many autistic students also find that they are particularly excited and interested by the academic challenge and intellectual stimulation of higher education, which helps to make the experience more enjoyable for them and increase their motivation.[22] For this to be the case, however, some students report it was especially important for them to align their chosen academic programs closely to their interests (Anderson et al., 2020).

By contrast, another motivating factor described by a number of students is, at least to some degree, spite. Many of the students interviewed across studies have had hurtful experiences in the past, either in university or in primary or secondary schooling, in which educators, peers, or others have expressed low expectations of them, or skepticism about their ability to succeed academically. The desire to prove those people wrong, or at least to prove themselves in general, was specifically mentioned as a powerful motivator by a number of students.[23] As one student in MacLeod et al. (2018) put it:

> Because I've got a lot of bad memories of people in education who basically said to my mum 'Josh will not achieve anything in his life'. And that's what drives you forward. It's like 'I will show you' and that's what it's all about really. (p. 690)

---

21 Melara, 2012; Tarallo, 2012; Ness et al., 2014; Bunch, 2016; Accardo et al., 2019b.
22 Ashby & Causton-Theoharis, 2012, Cullen, 2013; Drake, 2014; Anderson et al., 2017; Vincent et al., 2017; Ward & Webster, 2018.
23 Schaffer, 2013; Cipolla, 2018; Lambert & Dryer, 2018; MacLeod et al., 2018; Harn et al., 2019.

While of course the fact that so many students are able to transform these terrible experiences into a source of positive motivation is a demonstration of the courage and perseverance of these learners, it would be far preferable instead for them never to be subjected to such experiences at all. It is also worth noting that those who are not as able to overcome past emotional harm are no less worthy of the right to succeed in higher education.

Foundations of Identity and Confidence

Another valuable strength students report developing is the ability to thoroughly know, understand, and feel confident in themselves. Student self-awareness and metacognition have been linked with academic persistence across the literature on students with disabilities in higher education (Kutscher & Tuckwiller, 2019). Across an overwhelming number of narratives considered here, students are in agreement about the value of knowing their own strengths and weaknesses, how they best think and work, and how they most need to be supported.[24] In some cases, this was demonstrated to them negatively, by experiences of major struggle deriving from not being aware of their condition or their needs (Hubbard, 2011; Doikou-Avlidou, 2015; Lefler et al., 2016), and in others, students were able to gain significant insight into themselves through comparison to siblings and peers (Lux et al., 2016). In particular, a number of students particularly cite the importance of being aware of their individual strengths as well as weaknesses.[25] Developing positive self-acceptance of themselves, their characteristics, and their impairments is also mentioned by many students as critical to their success.[26]

Another factor that seems to support positive self-acceptance, as well as supporting student success in general, is a sense of positive disability identity: accepting and embracing that they are disabled, and that they would benefit from help and support in their areas of impairment, has

---

24   Heiney, 2011; Kirwan & Leather, 2011; Melara, 2012; Schaffer, 2013; Lux et al., 2016; Lightfoot et al., 2018; James et al., 2020.

25   Wilson, 2012; Doikou-Avlidou, 2015; Stampoltzis, 2015; Cipolla, 2018; Richardson, 2021.

26   Heiney, 2011; Kirwan & Leather, 2011; Carter & Sellman, 2013; Rutherford, 2013; Ennals et al., 2015; Brandt & McIntyre, 2016; Pfeifer et al., 2021.

repeatedly emerged from student interviews as a factor contributing to their success.[27] Along with self-acceptance in general, acceptance of a disabled identity can mitigate feelings of low academic self-confidence and not belonging in higher education, which can be frequent issues for students across many of these categories (Brandt & McIntyre, 2016). This is complicated, however, by the fact that students in these categories also tend to be less likely than other disabled students to accept their diagnoses and conditions, or to consider themselves to be disabled at all. Autistic and psychiatrically disabled students, in particular, appear to more often report ambivalence around whether they accept their respective diagnoses, and to be less likely to identify as disabled.[28] Acceptance of disability identity also tends to be complicated and uneven among chronically ill students, but especially crucial for success, as trying to push to imitate a nondisabled student's habits and patterns without support can in itself exacerbate illness symptoms and trigger health crises (Toller & Farrimond, 2021). These tendencies seem to contribute to the 'boom and bust' work pattern experienced by students who are mentally and physically chronically ill, as noted earlier: students assume that they do not need or do not deserve additional support, push themselves harder to succeed without it during periods of less severe symptoms, and by doing so trigger periods of more severe symptoms, which force them to reduce or stop their work again. A strong disability identity, meanwhile, seems to help facilitate more continuous support and balance, making these cycles less dramatic and disruptive.

While self-knowledge and self-confidence are consistently described as beneficial to students, however, it is also plain from students' narratives that these are skills that take time and effort to develop. Many students describe experiences of their capacity for self-understanding, acceptance, confidence, and advocacy gradually increasing over their time in college, as they matured and became more familiar with the college environment.[29] Older and more mature learners, such as

---

27 Erten, 2011; Heiney, 2011; Hubbard, 2011; Melara, 2012; Kreider et al., 2015; Sayman, 2015; Goodman, 2017; Clouder et al., 2020; James et al., 2020; Cox et al., 2021.

28 Simmeborn Fleischer, 2012; Downing, 2014; Kent, 2015; Sayman, 2015; Goodman, 2017; MacLeod et al., 2018; Cox et al., 2021.

29 Hubbard, 2011; Zafran et al., 2011; Ennals et al., 2015; Lux et al., 2016; Bolourian et al., 2018; Anderson et al., 2020; Cage & Howes, 2020; Grabsch et al., 2021.

returning students of nontraditional age, also appear to be more successful in college, likely because of similar factors (Bunch, 2016). It is heartening that students appear to be able to develop and strengthen these skills eventually, even if they are not present or strong at the start of higher education. As mentioned in the previous chapter, however, this means that students are likely to struggle much more early in college, and may fail, drop out, experience health crises, or some combination of these before they have time to learn the skills that would ultimately allow them to succeed. It could be beneficial to embed intentional coaching to support the development of these skills and attributes during the transition to university and in first-year support programs, or to strengthen it where it is already present.

Course Design and Student Needs

Overall Course Structure

Across a wide variety of student experiences, clear and coherent course organization overwhelmingly emerges as a valuable support—and the lack thereof as a significant barrier. Students with many different types of needs report that they particularly rely on strong course organization and structure to help them manage their academic work.[30] Careful structure, organization, and clarity are particularly important in online course environments, and when they are lacking, unfamiliar user interfaces and lack of context can make navigating the course at all an onerous, confusing challenge.[31] Course organization elements that have significant impacts include clear expectations for students, such as clearly communicated assignment instructions,[32] and clarity of course schedules and timelines (Redpath et al., 2013; Toor et al., 2016; Jansen et al., 2018). In poorly organized courses, students may find themselves unable to benefit from their own academic self-management and coping

---

30 Bush et al., 2011; Gelbar et al., 2015; Van Hees et al., 2015; Cai & Richdale, 2016; Toor et al., 2016; Anderson et al., 2018; Jansen et al., 2018; Cage & Howes, 2020; James et al., 2020; Maurer-Smolder et al., 2021.

31 Graves et al., 2011; Madaus et al., 2011; J.B. Roberts et al., 2011; Madaus et al., 2012; Catalano, 2014; Meyers & Bagnall, 2015.

32 Melara, 2012; Brazier, 2013; Rutherford, 2013; Cai & Richdale, 2016; White et al., 2016; Jansen et al., 2018; Gurbuz et al., 2019.

strategies, and may more easily become overwhelmed by their workload (James et al., 2020; Maurer-Smolder et al., 2021). Autistic students in one study explicitly wished for accommodations that would help them know what to expect from courses, such as priority access to course registration and advance knowledge of faculty office hours, to aid in managing their schedules (Accardo et al., 2019a).

To be clear, invisibly disabled and neurodivergent students do not need faculty to change the structure of each course to meet each student's individual preferences; this expectation would be not only unrealistic but unnecessary. What students need is for every course to have a thoughtful structure that is made explicitly clear, so that every student has as much advance knowledge as possible of what will be expected of them when and how, in order to plan for any potential problem areas. Even better, as indicated across a number of studies, is if the course and curriculum can be flexible, or modified when necessary, or both.[33] For example, across many student narratives, exams and other time-limited assessments emerge as a very common source of stress and accommodation need, especially when they are high-stakes, infrequent, inflexibly delivered, or any combination of these.[34] Rather than requiring students to invest significant additional time and effort into requesting and using special accommodations, faculty could instead consider permitting more flexibility in the time allotted for all students to complete tests. If specific time constraints are important for the skill to be tested, lower-stakes tests could at least be delivered more frequently throughout the term. In many cases, however, learning could very likely be evaluated with alternative types of assessment, which students who struggle in this area have indicated would be even more valuable (Erten, 2011; Kent, 2015; Gurbuz et al., 2019).

What appears to be most important is not the specifics of what faculty do to structure their courses, but that they clearly communicate their choices to students, and allow students as much control as possible over how they meet the requirements. In addition to aiding academic performance, supports that increase students' sense of

---

33 Gelbar et al., 2014; Van Hees et al., 2015; Cai & Richdale, 2016; Sarrett, 2017; Anderson et al., 2018; Ward & Webster, 2018; Lipka et al., 2019; Anderson et al., 2020.

34 Gelbar et al., 2014; Toor et al., 2016; Anderson et al., 2017; Smith, 2017; Anderson et al., 2018; Anderson et al., 2020; Clouder et al., 2020; Maurer-Smolder et al., 2021.

control over their coursework can significantly reduce the impact of anxiety disorders—sometimes to the point where, ironically, students no longer feel support is needed (Sokal & Desjardins, 2016). Another example of a beneficial strategy that increases students' sense of control is trigger warnings for sensitive course content (Orem & Simpkins, 2015). Sharing control of higher education experiences and helping to bolster students' confidence may seem like small gestures, but they can be uniquely powerful in their impacts.

Instructional Settings and Delivery

Another commonly recurring theme in students' narratives is that the physical environment of traditional lecture hall classrooms presents particular challenges. For example, traditional classrooms tend to foster many distractions, which is an issue given how common focus and attention challenges are as symptoms.[35] Noise and crowded spaces are also reported present slightly different challenges for autistic students, however, in the form of sensory overstimulation and heightened anxiety (Casement et al., 2017; Bolourian et al., 2018). Additionally, the size and configuration of lecture hall environments can increase students' difficulties with hearing and understanding professors, which is of significant concern for students who may already have language processing impairments (Mullins and Preyde, 2013). Smaller class sizes may help to mitigate these issues, regardless of course type (Hux et al., 2010; Melara, 2012; Lipka et al., 2019).

A traditional lecture style of teaching, similarly, can also be especially challenging for some students. Dyslexic students in several studies report difficulties with following class lectures (Clouder et al., 2020; Maurer-Smolder et al., 2021), as well as taking notes on them.[36] This is also true in many cases, however, of autistic students (Anderson et al., 2017; Accardo et al., 2019; Accardo et al., 2019b). On the whole, many students—especially those with ADHD and dyslexia—report benefiting most when instructors vary their instruction styles to be

---

35   Mullins & Preyde, 2013; Pirttimaa, 2015; Casement et al., 2017; Bolourian et al., 2018; Jones, 2020.

36   Olofsson et al., 2012; Pino & Mortari, 2014; Stampoltzis, 2015; MacCullagh et al., 2016; Smith, 2017; Clouder et al., 2020; Maurer-Smolder et al., 2021.

inclusive of different learning types and needs.[37] This includes in online instruction, where a number of students prefer interactive and hands-on learning exercises even in asynchronous online learning environments, over more passive formats like video (Catalano, 2014; Maurer-Smolder et al., 2021).

Methods of varying instructional delivery can take a number of beneficial forms. Across several studies, students with ADHD in particular felt they would benefit from interactivity and active engagement in the delivery of instruction, and also from information presented in multiple sensory formats, particularly visually (Heiney, 2011; Hubbard, 2011; Melara, 2012) Some students with ADHD also felt they would benefit most from instruction that includes repetition and reinforcement of information, opportunities for hands-on practice, and practical demonstrations of concepts (Lipka et al., 2019). Dyslexic students in Cipolla (2018) reported the most benefit from instructional activities that involved physical action and interaction, those that had a creative element, or both. In the same vein, in Clouder et al. (2020), students with both dyslexia and ADHD felt that interactive and otherwise nontraditional approaches to instruction were most helpful to them, while autistic students found that they received the most benefit from instruction that included a mentoring component and connections to practical application. Representing information in multiple sensory formats (visual, audio, etc.) has also been identified as valuable by autistic students, in cases where students have sensory processing issues with one or more formats (Ashby & Causton-Theoharis, 2012). As with course structure, it is not that there is one type of instruction that will most benefit neurodivergent and invisibly disabled learners, nor that every possible type of instruction needs to be included to cater to every possible preference. Instead, the more varied types of instruction are present, the better the chances of accommodating a greater variety of needs.

Much the same is true when it comes to the mode of instruction. Neither face-to-face instruction nor online is necessarily preferable for all categories, or even for all students within an individual category; autistic students, for example, report very mixed preferences across studies

---

37 Erten, 2011; Heiney, 2011; Hubbard, 2011; Flowers, 2012; Melara, 2012; Catalano, 2014; Smith, 2017; Sarrett, 2017; Cipolla, 2018; Lipka et al., 2019; Clouder et al., 2020; Maurer-Smolder et al., 2021; Richardson, 2021.

(Anderson et al., 2018; Lizotte, 2018; Adams et al., 2019). Some elements, however, can make each mode more or less helpful. Students in online courses can feel isolated from peers,[38] as well as from faculty (Madaus et al., 2011; Madaus et al., 2012; Adams et al., 2019), to the detriment of their learning experiences. Careful implementation, however, can make online course management systems a useful communication channel for students who would otherwise struggle to speak in class or to contact their instructors (Madaus et al., 2011; Madaus et al., 2012; Stampoltzis et al., 2015). Poor interface design in online learning systems can present major challenges for neurodivergent and invisibly disabled students,[39] such as a 'tunnel vision' effect some neurodivergent learners experience that causes them to hyperfocus on some interface elements and miss others (Meyers & Bagnall, 2015; Adams et al., 2019), or issues with cognitive load and information overload (Kent, 2015; Kent et al., 2018; Adams et al., 2019). Even so, the benefits of having course materials available online are significant,[40] as will be discussed in more detail next.

Course Materials

It is common for students in these categories to need access to course materials outside of class as an accommodation in general, whether these are notes, slides, or recordings, online or off. Being able to access instructional materials outside of class meetings provides a wide variety of affordances all at once, via the same relatively simple action: it enables review and re-study of material for students with attention and memory issues or who may need to be absent frequently; it provides control over playback and speed of recorded materials for those with sensory processing issues or impairments; it allows additional contact time with material for students with slower cognitive speeds; and more. What should be an easy accessibility win, however, in some cases proves complicated and frustrating for students instead.

While many students across studies express the need for course materials outside class, they also report varying rates of success in

---

38   Habib et al., 2012; Madaus et al., 2012; Heindel, 2014; Meyers & Bagnall, 2015; Adams et al., 2019.

39   Graves et al., 2011; Habib et al., 2012; Hollins & Foley, 2013; Downing, 2014; Kent et al., 2018; Adams et al., 2019.

40   Graves et al., 2011; Madaus et al., 2011; Madaus et al., 2012; Melara, 2012; Stampoltzis et al., 2015; Adams et al., 2019.

receiving them.[41] Some students indicate that the timing of when they receive course materials is also important: in most cases they require course materials before the actual class instruction period for these to be most helpful, and this need is not always met (Olofsson et al., 2012; Brazier, 2013; Toor et al., 2016). This is an area where online courses often provide superior affordances, as course materials are available at all times by default in this learning environment (Graves et al., 2011; Madaus et al., 2011, 2012). This effect can also be achieved, however, by consistent use of a course shell for face-to-face courses—provided, of course, that faculty are willing. A number of students also report that whether faculty actually provided course materials to them was often largely dependent on personality, with some responding to students' requests with reluctance or outright refusal (Stein, 2013; Strnadova et al., 2015). This is concerning, especially given that what faculty in these cases refuse to do—sharing material that would need to be prepared for class anyway—is arguably the simplest possible task to accommodate students' needs. This is not encouraging about faculty willingness to use more complicated and time-consuming methods of capturing class information, like recording class sessions.

Course Policies and Technology

Specific types of face-to-face course policies are frequently cited by students as another barrier to academic success. Required attendance policies, in particular, can present significant challenges for students across multiple categories of difference. Chronic illnesses can cause frequent absences for students, which already create issues for students academically, socially, and financially (where it affects them in the workplace), and these problems are only exacerbated by courses with strict attendance policies (Giroux et al., 2016; Barber & Williams, 2021). This is especially true in cases where faculty require medical documentation for absences, as in many cases not only does this documentation intrude on the privacy of students with chronic conditions, but it can also be difficult to procure, especially for students

---

41   Bush et al., 2011; Olofsson et al., 2012; Brazier, 2013; Gelbar et al., 2014; Pino & Mortari, 2014; Stampoltzis, 2015; Toor et al., 2016; MacCullagh et al., 2016; Anderson et al., 2018; Serry et al., 2018; Accardo et al., 2019a & 2019b; Anderson et al., 2020.

who have frequent and routine needs for medical care that disrupt their schedules (Barber & Williams, 2021). As indicated by Turosak and Siwierka (2021), however, students may also run afoul of attendance policies with any type of condition that impairs concentration or negatively affects rest and sleep—which are frequent symptoms of nearly all of the conditions under discussion here. While requiring class attendance may be intended to help students, by ensuring that they will be present to engage with course content alongside their peers, policies implemented without care and flexibility can be more harmful to students than they are helpful.

Another type of course policy that presents barriers to students is any policy restricting the use of technology in the classroom, particularly mobile phones and laptop computers (Pfeifer et al., 2021). These types of devices can be used to support assistive technologies for students with some types of conditions: for example, mobile devices or applications for reminders and scheduling can be particularly valuable to students with traumatic brain injuries and with chronic illnesses in general (Brown et al., 2017; Ravert et al., 2017; Leopold et al., 2019). Furthermore, students across multiple studies have indicated that general access to computing technology can act as a support for multiple conditions and ease relevant learning barriers.[42] Restricting students' access to technology in the classroom, therefore, although it is intended by faculty to reduce distractions, may instead deprive some students of tools that they rely on to help them maintain focus and manage their learning. As with attendance policies, while certain courses and situations may demand some limitation of the technological devices that are present, any policy along these lines should be implemented only with care, flexibility, and consideration for accessibility needs.

When available and used effectively, however, technology can be extremely helpful, and this is even true when the student in question cannot physically be present in the classroom at all. Students with chronic illnesses in particular are frequently forced to miss class sessions due to changes in their symptoms, but the option of providing hybrid or flexible class attendance using video conferencing and other technologies can help students to remain included and engaged even when they cannot be physically present (Giroux et al., 2016). Furthermore, due to the need

---

42   Hubbard, 2011; Bunch, 2016; Giroux et al., 2016; Grabsch et al., 2016.

for this type of flexibility during the isolation periods of the COVID-19 pandemic, far more faculty are now familiar with teaching this way than were at the study's time of writing, making this suggestion more feasible than ever to implement. Neither are chronically ill students the only ones in these categories for whom frequent absences are an issue. Students with psychiatric disabilities may also struggle to make class meeting times during periods of particular mental health struggle, and it could place less sensory stress on autistic students to attend classes remotely as needed. By effective use of technology, not only could the classroom environment be improved for students, it could be extended to include remote environments where students can have more of the affordances they need to be successful. This is only possible, however, if the student has the appropriate resources. A student without financial access to technology may not be able to access necessary tools unless provided with a computer, either in the classroom or—better still—by the institution as part of a one-to-one laptop program.

Summary and Conclusions

Negative experiences with higher education faculty and staff, especially teaching faculty, make up a concerningly common thread across student narratives. Some of the incidents described have significantly damaging impacts, both academically and psychologically. A large number of students report experiences of being misunderstood, dismissed, or belittled by faculty on divulging their support needs. These experiences are particularly frustrating because, when faculty are simply empathetic and supportive, the positive impacts of those experiences are similarly transformative. This raises questions of faculty accountability for their behavior toward this marginalized community, and how it affects students' learning environment. While fortunately the most severe mistreatment seems to be relatively rare, it is important for departments across the institution to be aware that it is still possible, and to take proactive steps to ensure that students are as protected as possible, and have transparent channels for addressing discrimination. In less serious cases, increased professional development and support for faculty would likely address many of students' concerns.

At the same time, students' academic lives are also impacted by internal factors. Across multiple categories, they are especially likely to struggle with aspects of information processing and communication, which disadvantages them in meeting common requirements of academic work. The invisibility of their conditions also presents challenges for students across all categories, making it more difficult for them to obtain necessary supports. In some cases, symptoms also fluctuate and cycle in unpredictable ways, creating further difficulties. On the other hand, many students find that they are able to develop self-knowledge, corresponding study strategies, and ways of motivating themselves, all of which benefit them significantly in their academic work. A sense of positive disability identity helps to foster all of these skills. Like all of these strategies, however, this tends to take time and maturation to develop, leaving students more at risk earlier in their college careers, and more so the less mentorship and support they have in developing in these directions.

This makes it all the more important to work toward designing and delivering more inclusive courses, which can begin from a few relatively simple actions. Clear, consistent, and organized course structure, with transparent instructions for assignments and assessments, provides a critical foundation for accommodating a wide variety of needs. Lecture-style teaching and classroom setups may be barriers for some students, but varying instruction styles and providing opportunities for interactivity can help mitigate these issues without necessarily changing an instructor's entire pedagogical approach. Online courses need to take particular care to avoid making students feel isolated, or overwhelming them with confusing and distracting elements. Simply providing lecture slides and notes for reference outside of class already improves the accessibility of a course significantly, leaving aside whether instructors can or will take the extra step of audio- or video-recording class instruction. Providing ample feedback, monitoring and guiding group work, and implementing course policies around attendance and technology with care, and only when necessary, will also eliminate many of the most significant barriers that vulnerable students face in the classroom.

If these recommendations sound like a simple matter of being a conscientious, attentive, and compassionate educator, it is because that is precisely what they are. The factors that make learning more manageable for neurodivergent and invisibly disabled students sometimes center around particular and even unexpected themes, but on the whole, they are not mysterious secrets. They are much the same factors that make a course more manageable for any student. As previously discussed, for that matter, neither is being neurodivergent or disabled a binary off-on switch. Each is a continuum, along which some students with more 'severe' challenges than others may nonetheless have strengths in the areas that allow them to be academically successful, and some students with 'milder' challenges may nonetheless have particular weaknesses that cause them to need significant help to succeed. Still other students may never have been diagnosed with any condition at all, for any number of reasons, and yet may have greater needs in certain areas than do students who have applied and qualified for formal accommodations. A rising tide of course accessibility will truly lift all boats, and meet more genuine needs than only those that have been presented with an accommodation letter. This, too, is one of the core principles behind Universal Design for Learning (UDL) as an approach.

Faculty, however, face their own barriers in making these changes. Instructors are frequently overextended and asked to do too much with too little, dividing their attention between teaching, research, and service requirements, and this tension tends to be especially acute for faculty with marginalized identities, including faculty who are disabled themselves. It may come as a major burden to ask them to exert additional efforts, without significant institutional support, to implement structural improvements to their courses, even if it is in order to make them more supportive for students. Unlike primary and secondary educators, also, higher education faculty are not universally taught pedagogical skills prior to undertaking teaching responsibilities. Training in this area is by no means a component of all doctoral programs to this day, and this is to say nothing of the many courses that are taught, especially in universities, by contingent faculty who may not have completed doctoral programs, and who are neither afforded enough control over the courses they teach nor compensated appropriately for the required time to be able to make substantive changes. Many institutions are also reluctant to impose any teaching standards or requirements on faculty with more time and security, in the name of academic freedom— including requirements affecting accessibility and student learning. Where this is the case, however, it is an erroneous application of the principle. Academic freedom is extremely valuable and of critical importance, but it concerns the protection of potentially controversial instructional content and methods, not the protection of faculty from accountability to their students for ethics and equity concerns. Clearer and more consistently applied expectations might well be of significant benefit not only for students, but for instructors also.

Similarly, in some cases faculty are hesitant to implement changes that might make courses easier for students, even if they might make the course easier for *all* students, for fear that this will compromise the course's rigor (Tobin & Behling, 2018, p. 35). This, too, is based on an erroneous assumption: the false equivalence of 'rigor' with 'difficulty,' or even with inflexibility specifically. This is a perception that Pfeifer et al. (2021) note is particularly prevalent in STEM fields. None of the course elements discussed in this chapter, however, would affect a course's rigor to modify, in that they would not compromise students' authentic learning of the course concepts. Students' success in a given course should not be measured on their ability to argue with faculty over whether they should receive accommodations, nor to navigate confusing course organization or guess at unclear structure and directions, nor to eschew technology, nor even to have perfect attendance. Flexibility in these matters decreases difficulty only in the *'how'* of learning, not in the *'what'*. Sometimes, certainly, it is necessary for a course to proceed in a certain way that requires specific logistical elements, or for students to learn course content under specific conditions. Even in those cases, however, there are likely to be ways that instructors can be transparent and deliberate about those needs, and even flexible within their parameters, without compromising the rigor of the course. It may simply require creativity, and the willingness to engage students as partners and collaborators.

5. Co-Curricular Campus Life

As important as the academic curriculum is, it is not the only important aspect of the higher education experience. Life on campus outside the classroom also has a significant impact on students' happiness, well-being, and academic success. A college or university is not just a place of learning, but also one where students socialize with each other, use spaces and facilities, and often reside. Often the academic and non-academic aspects of college life are not easily separated from one another, as well: examples include students' social relationships with peers in their courses, or their independent study arrangements outside of the classroom. Factors that affect neurodivergent and invisibly disabled students outside of class, positively or negatively, can have significant impacts on their academic lives, and the other way around.

Keeping in mind those complex interrelationships, this chapter will shift focus to common factors in student narratives that have their primary effects outside of the curriculum and classroom. These center around four main themes:

1. Social life and relationships with student peers, including social challenges;

2. Mental health challenges and needs;

3. Barriers and affordances in the physical environments of campus; and

4. Challenges and needs around daily living activities when residing on campus.

Many of the experiences discussed here focus on the challenges that invisibly disabled and neurodivergent students face in these areas. As in the previous chapter, however, in many cases they also point to affordances, actual and potential, that could improve students'

      https://doi.org/10.11647/OBP.0420.05

experiences in higher education and support their academic success. The seeds of these ideas will be expanded upon in greater detail, with examples of promising current practices, in the next section.

Social Life and Peer Relationships

Peer Relationships and Attitudes

Relationships with peers are tremendously important to students in college, and because of the nature of the university environment, they can affect almost every part of students' lives there: classes, socializing, athletics, living and dining arrangements, and more. Furthermore, positive relationships with peers are one of the most frequently cited forms of support upon which students rely, not only socially but for academic success and persistence as well.[1] Student narratives also report that socializing and maintaining a healthy personal life helps to support their well-being and mental health.[2] As is discussed elsewhere, this is an area of concern for students across all categories of difference, not only those specifically with psychiatric disabilities, so this type of support is particularly valuable. Some students, autistic students most frequently, report especially wanting and appreciating relationships with other disabled and neurodivergent peers.[3] Students in Cullen (2013) also describe establishing supportive social relationships with others online through social networks. In addition to their informal support networks of friends and classmates, a number of students also value more formal support from designated or volunteered academic support peers,[4] and peer support groups.[5]

---

1   Demery et al., 2012; Melara, 2012; Young, 2012; Cullen, 2013; Houman & Stapley, 2013; Rutherford, 2013; Schaffer, 2013; Schindler & Kietz, 2013; Pino & Mortari, 2014; Ennals et al., 2015; Kreider et al., 2015; Strnadova et al., 2015; Childers & Hux, 2016; Lux, 2016; Sokal & Desjardins, 2016; Casement et al., 2017; LeGary, 2017; Smith, 2017; Berry, 2018; Lightfoot et al., 2018; Accardo et al., 2019b; Davis, 2019; Kutscher & Tuckwiller, 2019; Winberg et al., 2019; Anderson et al., 2020; Giroux et al., 2020; Cox et al., 2021; Pfeifer et al., 2021; Turosak & Siwierka, 2021.
2   Zafran et al., 2011; LeGary, 2017; Smith, 2017; Turosak & Siwierka, 2021.
3   Cullen, 2013; Schwenk et al., 2014; Accardo et al., 2019b; Anderson et al., 2020.
4   Randolph, 2012; Strnadova et al., 2015; Ravert et al., 2017; Kutscher & Tuckwiller, 2019.
5   Erten, 2011; Cullen, 2013; Houman & Stapley, 2013; Anderson et al., 2017; Sarrett, 2017; Serry et al., 2018; Accardo et al., 2019b; Hoffman et al., 2019; Anderson et al., 2020; Giroux et al., 2020; Grabsch et al., 2021.

As with faculty, however, the support that friends and other peers are able to provide in positive relationships makes negative experiences with peers all the more painful. Not only does this mean an experience of hurtful social rejection, but also that students miss out on potential benefits to their lives in college. Students' narratives in some studies also suggest that negative experiences of ableism by peers can have other damaging effects, including discouraging students from seeking more formal support (Winberg et al., 2019; Lett et al., 2020; Pfeifer et al., 2021). For example, one student described being discouraged by an experience with a classmate:

> She said [students who use accommodations] are not on the same playing field as everyone else [because they use accommodations]. I said, "No, I actually have this diagnosed thing. Here's a report on it." And she was like, "Well, yeah, a lot of people get diagnosed with ADHD." (Pfeifer et al., 2021, p. 9)

It should come as no surprise, therefore, that students across many studies report being reluctant or afraid to disclose a disability or neurodivergence to peers, due to concern about stigmatizing responses or other misperceptions and negative reactions.[6] In some other cases, students may prefer to be open with peers from the beginning, to get the process of disclosure out of the way and provide clarity (Knott & Taylor, 2014; Lizotte, 2018). It could be argued, however, that this is also a way of managing anxieties around disclosure.

Neither are those anxieties unfounded. Many student narratives describe lived experiences of stigma and negative attitudes from peers on disclosing a neurodivergence or invisible disability.[7] In Doikou-Avlidou (2015), dyslexic students in Greek universities describe experiencing so much social stigma that they became isolated from their peers. In other cases, even among friends and otherwise understanding peers, a number of students describe experiences of peers expressing skepticism about their needs, such as accusations or implications of 'faking it' (Young, 2012; Gottschall & Young, 2017). Others describe peers expressing

---

6   Zafran et al., 2011; Demery et al., 2012; Simmeborn Fleischer, 2012; Schwenk et al., 2014; Ennals et al., 2015; Van Hees et al., 2015; Giroux et al., 2016; Casement et al., 2017; Hadley, 2017; Lightfoot et al., 2018; Giroux et al., 2020; Miller et al., 2020.

7   Heiney, 2011; Doikou-Avlidou, 2015; Gelbar et al., 2015; Pirttimaa, 2015; Timmerman & Mulvihill, 2015; Gottschall & Young, 2017; Lightfoot et al., 2018; VanderLind, 2018; Kain et al., 2019.

resentment of their accommodations, and in particular of ADHD medication, as supposedly unfair advantages.[8] Avoiding disclosure, however, is not always a preferable solution, as some students report that their efforts to hide their disability or neurodivergence led to feeling poorly understood and isolated.[9] Masking symptoms of a condition or neurodivergent behaviors can also be a source of stress in itself, such as for students with Ehlers-Danlos syndrome in Giroux et al. (2016). Being open with peers can come at a social cost for students, but so, clearly, can secrecy. Both choices can compromise the informal support networks that so many students report are beneficial.

Social Challenges

To make matters worse, other social challenges are also common for invisibly disabled and neurodivergent students. This is true across multiple categories, but they tend to be especially commonly reported by autistic students. Across an overwhelming number of studies, autistic students describe feelings of difference from others in college, and a sense of both desire and inability to 'fit in'.[10] In some cases, these difficulties have been exacerbated by their peers' misunderstandings, ignorance, or stigmatizing of autism—or the fear that they will do so if the student's identity becomes known.[11] Several students across studies report having been bullied, either prior to or in college,[12] although others report higher education has been a much safer environment from bullying than secondary education was (Anderson et al., 2018).

Indeed, the biggest challenges for autistic students seem to be in finding common ground with their undergraduate peers, and some

---

8   Young, 2012; Mullins & Preyde, 2013; Kreider et al., 2015; Gottschall & Young, 2017; Pfeifer et al., 2021.

9   Erten, 2011; Ennals et al., 2015; Casement et al., 2017; Miller et al., 2020.

10   Madriaga, 2010; Simmeborn Fleischer, 2012; Simmeborn Fleischer, 2013; Rutherford, 2013; Drake, 2014; Gelbar et al., 2014; Knott & Taylor, 2014; Strnadova et al., 2015; Van Hees et al., 2015; Anderson et al., 2017; Casement et al., 2017; LeGary, 2017; Vincent et al., 2017; Bolourian et al., 2018; Jansen et al., 2018; Ward & Webster, 2018; Harn et al., 2019; Anderson et al., 2020; Cage & Howes, 2020; Clouder et al., 2020.

11   Gelbar et al., 2014; Casement et al., 2017; Vincent et al., 2017; Winberg et al., 2019.

12   Simmeborn Fleischer, 2012; Cullen, 2013; Winberg et al., 2019; Krumpelman & Hord, 2021.

report finding it easier to form connections with faculty (Accardo et al., 2019a). Not only do students struggle with establishing social connections in general, furthermore, but some report specific difficulties with forming deep friendships (Cullen, 2013) and romantic relationships (Colclough, 2018). As a result of all of these factors, many autistic students describe feeling lonely and isolated, but pulled between wanting social connections and the relative safety and ease of remaining alone.[13] Not only do autistic students express personal desire to connect, as well, but they also explicitly recognize in some interviews that they are lacking social support networks that would be beneficial in managing stress and academic challenges (White et al., 2016; Ward & Webster, 2018). Even so, their experiences of being made to feel different and ostracized can make reaching out to others seem not worth the risk. As a student in Vincent et al. (2017) poignantly described, "I want to socialise and have friends like any normal people, but every time the invitation comes, I almost always go into default mode and say 'no'" (p. 309).

Another source of significant academic and social challenges for autistic students, as well, is lack of acceptance in university of idiosyncratic behavior and movements often characteristic of autistic people, such as stimming (Sarrett, 2017; Jansen et al., 2018). Stigma against these characteristics can result not only in exacerbated social difficulties, but in students' being judged negatively in academic settings, and most often pressure falls on autistic students to disguise themselves and conform to neurotypical expectations, rather than on peers and faculty to accept them as they are. For example, some students describe experiences where they sought out supports that would relieve their academic stress and challenges, but found that university staff instead prioritized 'fixing' their social skills to align more with neurotypical behavior (Cage & Howes, 2020). As discussed, positive disability identity and self-acceptance are of great importance to student success and well-being, but students find it difficult to accept themselves when they are asked

---

13   Madriaga, 2010; Simmeborn Fleischer, 2012; Tarallo, 2012; Cullen, 2013; Gelbar et al., 2014; Gelbar et al., 2015; Sayman, 2015; Van Hees et al., 2015; Toor et al., 2016; Casement et al., 2017; Vincent et al., 2017; Anderson et al., 2018; Bolourian et al., 2018; Ward & Webster, 2018; Gurbuz et al., 2019; Harn et al., 2019; Anderson et al., 2020; Cage & Howes, 2020; Krumpelman & Hord, 2021.

to repress their natural behaviors in order to facilitate social interactions (Cox et al., 2017). Masking autistic behaviors is common for students, but it is also intensely exhausting and stressful (Anderson et al., 2020; Cox et al., 2021). All of the various pressures to mimic neurotypical behavior also compound the significant stress that autistic students experience, from academics and from the unfamiliar and unpredictable environmental factors that they have particular difficulty managing, and stress can compound these students' existing behavioral challenges and difficulties with managing emotions (Brazier, 2013; White et al., 2016). In combination with other pressures, the pressure to suppress minor and benign behaviors can actually contribute to outbursts and meltdowns that are much more disruptive—for the autistic student at least as much as for those around them. Fostering an aware, compassionate, accepting environment would be the more beneficial priority, rather than pushing autistic students to change for the comfort of others.

Social challenges have a large impact on students with psychiatric disabilities as well as autistic students, albeit usually for different reasons. As previously mentioned, because of the significant stigma around psychiatric disabilities, these students frequently describe experiencing feelings of shame and guilt about their conditions, and a perceived need to keep them secret.[14] These concerns impact students' reaching out for support services, of course, but may also take such personal forms as students internalizing stigma and feeling 'broken' (VanderLind, 2018). As a result of these and other factors, students with psychiatric disabilities often report feeling isolated and in need of more social support;[15] having low self-esteem related to shame about their symptoms and academic challenges (Hubbard, 2011; Sokal & Desjardins, 2016); and avoiding social contact, whether out of distrust, fear of discovery, or vulnerability if others learn more about them.[16] Isolation is also reported by student veterans with trauma disorders, as, due to their military service, they are often at a different stage of life and maturity than traditional college students (Ness et al., 2014). For other students, substance abuse issues and the need to avoid triggering situations can

---

14 Hubbard, 2011; Demery et al., 2012; Stein, 2013; Sokal & Desjardins, 2016.
15 Hubbard, 2011; Demery et al., 2012; Sokal & Desjardins, 2016; Winberg et al., 2019; Miller et al., 2020.
16 Demery et al., 2012; Markoulakis & Kirsh, 2013; Ennals et al., 2015; Sokal & Desjardins, 2016; VanderLind, 2018; Winberg et al., 2019.

further limit socializing options on campus, where alcohol and other substances are likely to be prevalent (Demery et al., 2012). All of these anecdotal experiences are corroborated by the broader data, which show that students with psychiatric disabilities are less likely than others to participate in social activities and events, and to individually meet with faculty when not required (Koch et al., 2014). As alluded to earlier, this tendency is of particular concern for this population, as students who have experienced a mental health crisis specifically identify social connections and personal life balance as important factors in restoring and maintaining mental health (Zafran et al., 2011).

In general, autistic and psychiatrically disabled students seem to report the most social challenges, and the significant overlap between these two groups may concentrate these factors. Social challenges are also present, however, for students in other categories. Some students with ADHD, for example, describe difficulties with interpersonal relationships, including trouble with emotional outbursts and struggling to form deep friendships (Kwon et al., 2018). Social issues are also not uncommon for students with TBI: several narratives describe factors that affect students socially, such as finding that they are not able to participate in the same activities and hobbies that had previously been a foundation for social relationships, or that others or they themselves feel that they are 'not the same person' anymore (Bush et al., 2011; Gottschall & Young, 2017; Davis, 2019). A student's sense of identity may be in transition after a brain injury, an emotional journey that can be difficult and isolating, and can make connecting with others more challenging (Gottschall & Young, 2017; Davis, 2019). A number of students with TBI also describe struggles with mood issues, including more negative and changeable emotions than average (Ness et al., 2014; Childers & Hux, 2016), as well as frustration and anger with their cognitive changes (Owens, 2020), which may impact their relationships with others. Some also report feeling that it takes more energy for them to be active socially than it has in the past (Childers & Hux, 2016), and others find it helpful to have social connections facilitated by structures like dedicated communities and programs (Leopold et al., 2019). This desire echoes similar needs for facilitated social interaction expressed by autistic students, as well.

Although social challenges appear to be less acute for chronically ill students, some do find that illness can cause them to feel different and socially isolated among other college students (Schwenk et al., 2014), and that having to manage the challenges of their health can be harmful to relationships (Barber & Williams, 2021). Students in some studies reported masking and hiding their conditions (Giroux et al., 2016; Barber & Williams, 2021), which can lead to feeling further isolated and less understood, as well as being a source of day-to-day emotional stress for the student (Giroux et al., 2016). Even when a student's condition is known, for that matter, they may experience negative, ableist, and unsympathetic responses from both faculty and peers (Hoffman et al., 2019; Giroux et al., 2020), and the unpredictable cycling of symptoms and needs that chronically ill students tend to experience makes it difficult to make and commit to social plans (Giroux et al., 2020). Some activities that might otherwise support students' forming social connections, like athletics, are also frequently out of reach for chronically ill students, when insufficient support is available for them to be confident in participating (Schwenk et al., 2014). It is significantly more difficult to form friendships when the spaces and programs where students most often socialize are not accessible to all.

Mental Health Challenges

Perhaps relatedly, students across many of the categories discussed here describe struggles with mental health concerns, which appear to be frequently linked to all relevant conditions, and which compound their challenges. Anxiety and depression are the most commonly experienced, and apart from students with psychiatric disabilities, they have been reported in larger numbers of autistic students than other categories.[17] Anxiety, however, is also fairly common among students with ADHD[18] and dyslexic students (Cameron, 2016; Lambert & Dryer, 2018; Clouder et al., 2020). Depression is also sometimes reported by students with ADHD (Bolourian et al., 2018; Clouder et al., 2020), dyslexic students (Clouder et al., 2020), and chronically ill students (Giroux et al., 2020).

---

17 Gelbar et al., 2014; Knott & Taylor, 2014; Gelbar et al., 2015; Van Hees et al., 2015; Cai & Richdale, 2016; Toor et al., 2016; White et al., 2016; Anderson et al., 2017; Anderson et al., 2018; Bolourian et al., 2018; Jansen et al., 2018; Ward & Webster, 2018; Accardo et al., 2019b; Gurbuz et al., 2019; Anderson et al., 2020; Clouder et al., 2020; Krumpelman & Hord, 2021.

18 Flowers, 2012; Melara, 2012; Bolourian et al., 2018; Kwon et al., 2018; Clouder et al., 2020.

Concurrent obsessive-compulsive disorder is less common, but also noted among students with ADHD (Melara, 2012) and autistic students (Cai & Richdale, 2016), while substance abuse issues have been noted by some chronically ill students (Barber & Williams, 2021). Anderson and Butt (2017) also note that in some cases, new or worsened mental health symptoms might be triggered by the transition to university.

Furthermore, even students without specific conditions also experience struggles related to mental health. Stress and overwhelm are frequently noted by students with ADHD, autistic students, chronically ill students, and dyslexic students.[19] Autistic students also appear to experience high stress and a low tolerance for stress, particularly when it comes to academic stressors.[20] Psychiatrically disabled students in Demery et al. (2012) note a particular need for stress management tools and structures, as well. Elevated rates of sleep disturbances and associated fatigue, which are intimately intertwined with mental health struggles, have also been noted by students across every category examined.[21] Where mental health challenges exist, furthermore, students report that they may be exacerbated by stigma and ableist microaggressions (Lett et al., 2020), as well as by struggles with disability needs and accommodations (Cai & Richdale, 2016).

> Student: I've had a screaming fit in the middle of the corridor at the admin building. My particular lecturer walked away from me when I asked for help and I said, don't you walk away. And I really lost it (Cai & Richdale, 2016, p. 36).

On a related note, chronically ill students describe a number of emotional impacts from their illnesses, in addition to the physical effects, and often caused by them. Some describe living with an illness as an 'emotional roller coaster' (Giroux et al., 2020), and having to manage not only symptoms but feelings of stress and frustration with how symptoms impact them (Giroux et al., 2016; Giroux et al., 2020), as well as feelings of lack of control over their lives (Schwenk et al.,

---

19 Melara, 2012; Tarallo, 2012; Cullen, 2013; Hughes et al., 2016; Lambert & Dryer, 2018; Clouder et al., 2020.

20 Simmeborn Fleischer, 2013; White et al., 2016; LeGary, 2017; Anderson et al., 2018; Berry, 2018; Jansen et al., 2018; Ward & Webster, 2018; Gurbuz et al., 2019; Anderson et al., 2020; Cage & Howes, 2020.

21 Schaffer, 2013; Simmeborn Fleischer, 2013; Ness et al., 2014; Childers & Hux, 2016; Anderson et al., 2018; Lambert & Dryer, 2018; Hoffman et al., 2019.

2014). On the other hand, an unexpected positive aspect some students have noted of having to manage their health carefully is that it can increase their awareness and caution against common reckless college behaviors, such as excessive drinking (Schwenk et al., 2014). Especially given these students' generally elevated stress levels, however, some note a consequent need for safer, more inclusive campus-provided opportunities for recreation and relaxation (Ravert et al., 2017).

Even beyond the obvious concerns about students' quality of life, these increased mental health challenges have other demonstrated effects as well. Mental health notably impacts academic performance (Goodman, 2017), and this effect is likely to be compounded by the other challenges facing invisibly disabled and neurodivergent students. For example, autistic students in Anderson et al. (2020) cite poor mental health as a major factor in higher education non-completion. As noted by participants in Turosak and Siwierka (2021), there is also reason to suspect that mental health issues on college campuses are more prevalent than is believed—which is concerning given how widespread these challenges are already believed to be.

For psychiatrically disabled students in particular, of course, there are other specific concerns around mental health. Perhaps the greatest of these is what Miller et al. (2020) describe as 'stacking stressors': the academic, mental health, and other challenges (such as, in the study by Miller et al., foster care experiences) that students encounter not only combine but compound each other in their effects on students' stress levels.[22] For example, not only are students' mental health symptoms problematic in themselves, but they have significant detrimental effects on their academic work, such as difficulties with concentration and motivation, and this increases academic stress as well.[23] Furthermore, even symptoms that do not directly affect students academically may do so indirectly, such as by impacting self-esteem, stress management, and self-care.[24] Experiences related to other illnesses and marginalized identities can also be compounding factors in students' stress levels, as well as triggers of trauma (Orem & Simpkins, 2015; Goodman, 2017; Conley et al., 2019).

---

22 Hubbard, 2011; Markoulakis & Kirsh, 2013; Ennals et al., 2015; Miller et al., 2020.
23 Markoulakis & Kirsh, 2013; Schindler & Kietz, 2013; Ennals et al., 2015; Kain et al., 2019; Jones, 2020; Turosak & Siwierka, 2021.
24 Markoulakis & Kirsh, 2013; Schindler & Kietz, 2013; Kent, 2015; Turosak & Siwierka, 2021.

These are not challenges that are unique to students with psychiatric disabilities, of course, but there is evidence that the higher education environment is more disabling for them than for others in relation to these issues (Markoulakis & Kirsh, 2013; McEwan & Downie, 2013). Students with psychiatric disabilities are less likely to graduate college even than students with other types of disabilities, and not because of poorer academic skills (Markoulakis & Kirsh, 2013; McEwan & Downie, 2013), as studies have indicated that their average grade performance is on par with the general population (Schindler & Kietz, 2013; Ness et al., 2014). Rather, these students are simply more likely to be at a significant disadvantage, which they may not fully understand or even recognize. The narratives of students with psychiatric disabilities often reflect a tendency to internalize their conditions as personal failings, to be overcome individually and secretly, rather than impairments others do not have to bear and that merit support and understanding. This tends to lead to significant negative impacts on self-esteem and feelings of shame and alienation.[25] Exacerbating these factors is the fact that psychiatrically disabled students may also experience cognitive distortions that impact their capacity for self-understanding, making it more difficult to conceptualize and quantify their experience, and making the aforementioned benefits of metacognition more difficult for them to access (Zafran et al., 2011; Jones, 2020). Students may not be able to easily recognize the impact their symptoms have on their academic work (Ness et al., 2014), and may be more inclined to believe and internalize incidences where others minimize their illness, due to lack of trust in their own perceptions (Turosak & Siwierka, 2021). As a result, students are less likely to seek the supports or take the precautions that they need to protect their well-being, and more likely to try to push through without acknowledging their impairments instead, which in many cases leads to a recurring pattern of decline, crisis, despair, and recovery (Ennals et al., 2015). As one might expect, if a student experiences an acute break or other mental health crisis in the course of their education, it creates a major disruption in every aspect of their lives, not to mention that these crises tend to be preceded by academic decline and failures that create additional stress for students to handle

---

25   Hubbard, 2011; Markoulakis & Kirsh, 2013; Sokal & Desjardins, 2016; VanderLind, 2018; Miller et al., 2020.

during their recovery period (Zafran et al., 2011). In this area as in many others, prevention would be far preferable to cure.

Campus Environments

Navigating the physical environment of campus may not present as many challenges for these categories of students as it does for those with sensory or mobility impairments, but it does present some. Specific groups such as autistic students or chronically ill students, in particular, commonly report unique needs that extend to their physical surroundings. This is especially true on a college or university campus, where many students not only attend classes but also study independently, socialize, eat meals, and reside in a shared living space. As an environment, college is one that students may occupy for more concentrated time than any other single place in their lives, and if it is a hostile environment for a student with unique needs, then it can be inescapably so.

General Concerns

There are a few concerns around spaces that apply generally across campus, rather than being specific to any one type of space. One is the need for access to transportation, both to and within campus, and issues with the distance, size, and navigability of campus itself. Autistic students in Anderson et al. (2020), for example, identify transportation help as one of their most desirable supports, with the implication being that transportation is one of many cumulative stressors around logistics and self-management that are particularly acute for these students, and any one of them is helpful to alleviate. Students in many categories may also have significantly greater need for medical care and supplies to be accessible on campus, such as prescription medications, but this is particularly true of chronically ill students (Ravert et al., 2017). Availability and privacy of bathroom facilities in all areas of campus can also be a significant issue across multiple types of conditions, especially chronic illness, and especially for illnesses that involve bowel dysfunction, which is one of the more common types of chronic illness that affects this age group (Schwenk et al., 2014). Any challenges with ready access to sufficiently private bathrooms may also be compounded for transgender and gender-nonconforming students, which is a population that has been found to notably overlap with neurodivergent students. Depending on the campus and its social climate, finding a public restroom they can use comfortably and without fear for their safety may already be a challenge for these students, and a related impairment can only make this more difficult.

Additional considerations around spaces are especially important for autistic students. Because of sensory sensitivities that are common for these students, campus environments with large amounts of noise or other sensory input can present barriers to their use of the space. If these factors are not considered and carefully managed, campus events, spaces, and even classrooms can be prohibitively inaccessible to autistic students.[26] In fact, some former students in Anderson et al. (2020) cite these types of issue as a significant factor in their degree non-completion. Carving out dedicated sensory-friendly spaces in academic buildings is of value to autistic students (Sarrett, 2017; Anderson et al., 2020), as well as in some cases to students with TBI who may have developed sensitivity to light and sound (Ness et al., 2014). Nonetheless, if noise and sensory input levels remain extremely high in other parts of campus that are necessary for students to navigate on a regular basis, many autistic students will still be at a severe disadvantage. At the same time, carefully designed campus environments may be able to help mitigate another challenge autistic students often report: difficulty with adaptation to the university environment, and with lack of consistency and structure in the college experience.[27] Carefully structuring the class, living, and social environments to provide consistency and stability, communicate expectations, and relieve sensory stress could be helpful in managing a number of these struggles.

---

26 Madriaga, 2010; Van Hees et al., 2015; Cai & Richdale, 2016; Anderson et al., 2017; Vincent et al., 2017; Anderson et al., 2018; Bolourian et al., 2018; Colclough, 2018; Jansen et al., 2018; Lizotte, 2018; Gurbuz et al., 2019; Winberg et al., 2019; Anderson et al., 2020; Cage & Howes, 2020.

27 Brazier, 2013; Van Hees et al., 2015; Cai & Richdale, 2016; Vincent et al., 2017; Bolourian et al., 2018; Jansen et al., 2018; Anderson et al., 2020; Cage & Howes, 2020; Grabsch et al., 2021; Krumpelman & Hord, 2021.

Living Environments

Additional concerns arise from the fact that many students do not only attend classes and study on campus, but live there as well. One issue that particularly impacts many autistic students is the incompatibility of on-campus living environments, particularly dormitory environments, with their individual needs. Many autistic students across studies describe struggling to share living space with others, whether for reasons of social discomfort with roommates and being in close proximity to so many other students,[28] sensitivity to overwhelming sensory input like noise and smells,[29] or both. Students in Accardo et al. (2019a) specifically identify accommodations in housing as a necessary support for these reasons, and those in Grabsch et al. (2021) also point to a need for outreach about accommodations that are available, to increase students' awareness of them.

For chronically ill students, dorm life and other on-campus living situations also often lack needed affordances for managing their conditions and treatments. For example, dormitories generally lack adequate access to refrigeration for important medications that require it (Schwenk et al., 2014; Hoffman et al., 2019). As previously mentioned, the issue of bathroom access and privacy discussed in Schwenk et al. (2014) can also be particularly acute in dormitory living environments, depending on the design and availability of the facilities. In addition, students with inflammatory bowel disease also frequently need careful dietary management for their conditions, which can be prohibitively difficult to maintain when using campus dining hall facilities (Schwenk et al., 2014).

Third Places

Beyond their classrooms and living environments, students also report environmental challenges in social and independent study spaces around campus. Environments like academic libraries, student centers, and computer labs can be just as important to students' success and well-being in college as the places where they attend classes and reside, and

---

28   Drake, 2014; Gelbar et al, 2014; Toor et al., 2016; Bolourian et al., 2018; Grabsch et al., 2021.

29   Knott & Taylor, 2014; Toor et al., 2016; Casement et al., 2017; Bolourian et al., 2018; Grabsch et al., 2021.

just as fraught with complications for those who are invisibly disabled and neurodivergent. This is of greatest concern for higher education staff, however, around spaces where students study and complete academic work.

Overall, the most common needs students describe for these spaces involve control of their environment, if only in individual study areas within a larger space. In particular, students need control of the level of privacy, noise, and ambient distraction where they are working. Being able to minimize distractions in their study environment is often mentioned as a significant need for students with TBI (Bush et al., 2011; Gottschall & Young, 2017; Owens, 2020), and, as one might expect, for students with ADHD (Hubbard, 2011; Schaffer, 2013). Noise control and the availability of quiet spaces is also of value for autistic students, as part of the value of sensory-friendly spaces in general (Anderson et al., 2020). Paradoxically, however, autistic students in other studies have also found shared spaces that are traditionally 'quiet spaces' on campus, such as college libraries, can be *too* quiet for them to be able to focus and study comfortably. A communal space like a library that is designated for quiet study, or even a shared quiet study room within a building, can make autistic students feel hypervisible and anxious about conforming to social expectations, especially with regard to autistic behaviors and movement like stimming (Madriaga, 2010; Anderson, 2018; Pionke et al., 2019). Access to secluded, private study spaces with control of noise and other sensory input, to reduce both distractions and self-conscious discomfort, is therefore a very helpful support for autistic students, even within otherwise quiet shared environments (Madriaga, 2010; Anderson, 2018; Pionke et al., 2019).

Pionke's (2017) study of university library accessibility yielded several additional insights into student needs in academic libraries, which may also have implications for other campus buildings. Students in the study note the importance of building cleanliness, which is a potential consideration for students in several of the categories here, as well as attention to multiple types of accessibility in the building's affordances and safety features. The importance of training and empathy for those who staff the building, with regard to the potential diverse needs of users, was also stressed. Helpful and thorough signage has been reported as another critical factor for students with multiple types of impairment (Everhart and Escobar, 2018). Finally, to ensure all of these factors and more are adequately addressed, Pionke (2017) indicates the importance of feedback mechanisms on spaces by which students and other users can convey any concerns.

When neurodivergent and invisibly disabled students struggle with the environment of study spaces, intersectional identities can also impact and exacerbate their challenges. For example, in Cameron and Greenland (2021), female students of color with dyslexia describe multiple layers of challenge in completing their work in university spaces, as opposed to their own personal residential spaces. Not only did university spaces lack tools and affordances that they needed to manage their study needs, and would have access to at home, but they were also adversely affected by trying to work in a STEM environment that was white- and male-dominated in terms of demographic makeup, expectations, and configuration. As the authors describe it:

> Riya's [one of the students interviewed] experience in university spaces appeared to be shaped by a number of different intersecting characteristics; the departmental learning spaces were populated by mostly white, mostly male, and mostly highly socio-economically privileged students; the course required high productivity, adherence to tight deadlines, and it nurtured peer-competition; being 'worldly', confident, and well-off appeared to be necessary for success (p. 76).

Riya and other disabled, female STEM students of color, they argue, may be made uncomfortable to the point of avoiding campus spaces where they are very visibly different and struggle to meet common social norms and expectations, and this is to their detriment. Particularly in STEM disciplines, there is a need for students to be able to utilize spaces like labs and computing spaces for specialized software, and not all work can feasibly be completed in the student's home. Facing intersectional barriers like these in university spaces is to the detriment of students' academic success and personal well-being.

Furthermore, improvements to existing campus spaces are not the only need that has been identified. Across a number of studies and categories, students also express a need for specifically neurodiversity- and disability-oriented social and study spaces on campus. Students mention that it would be helpful to have a dedicated workspace for their needs with a variety of different affordances, including a distraction-free environment (Hubbard, 2011), sensory-friendly facilities and practices by staff (Sarrett, 2017; Anderson et al., 2020), other supports for the environmental needs of neurodivergent and disabled students

(Scheef, 2019; Winberg et al., 2019), and associated availability of childcare while using these spaces (Hubbard, 2011). The most commonly mentioned factor students want from these types of spaces, however, is the opportunity to form communities with other disabled and neurodivergent students, including both informal social groups and formal support groups.[30] A disability- and neurodiversity-friendly communal campus space would ideally be able to perform a dual role in this respect, both facilitating structured social groups and providing opportunities for serendipitous meetings of similar peers.

Daily Living on Campus

In addition to the factors around living environments described above, how students manage the activities of daily living while residing on campus is another important matter, and one that is often under-addressed. Depending on a student's particular areas of impairment and their severity, neurodivergent and invisibly disabled students may need substantial support with these activities, particularly within their residential environment. This is especially true if they are newly living away from home and family for the first time, and needing to adjust to completing independently tasks with which they may always have had help in the past. Autistic students across studies, for example, particularly report struggling with tasks like cleaning, attending to personal hygiene, and remembering appointments (Simmeborn Fleischer, 2012; Simmeborn Fleischer, 2013; Toor et al., 2016). Students across multiple categories in Kreider et al. (2015) also express frustration with the time and academic impacts of managing daily living tasks that are not as well supported as academic needs. Depending on the level of severity of the injury, as well, TBI may carry more risk of significantly reducing students' independent functioning than some other conditions. TBI survivors in Bush et al. (2011) required substantial help from family and faculty to continue their academic studies, as well as other life activities, raising concerns about what becomes of the needs of students who have less support available.

---

30 Sokal & Desjardins, 2016; Sarrett, 2017; Vincent et al., 2017; Scheef, 2019; Winberg et al., 2019.

Summary and Conclusions

Socializing in university is a great source of enjoyment, stress relief, and restoration for many students, and respite during what can sometimes be a very challenging period of their lives. It can also, however, be extremely fraught and difficult for students in these categories. Friends and other student peers are a frequent source of vital support, but stigma, skepticism, and resentment are recurring obstacles to those positive relationships. Compounding this is that students with some conditions also struggle to develop relationships and social connections, which has an impact not only on their quality of life in college but on the informal supports that are available. These struggles are particularly acute for autistic and psychiatrically disabled students, but are also present across other categories. All students, across all categories, are also at increased risk of mental health challenges. These may take the form of psychiatric disabilities, such as anxiety or depression, or more rarely conditions like obsessive-compulsive disorder, substance abuse disorders, or others. They may also take the form of more common experiences like stress, overwhelm, and sleep disturbances. Mental health symptoms can be exacerbated by the other disability-related challenges that students face, and have significant impacts on well-being and academic success.

At the same time, there are other supports and challenges for students in the campus environment. In general, students need reliable and discreet access to transportation, medical supplies, and bathroom facilities to be able to manage a variety of conditions, regardless of where they are on campus. Campus spaces can also present specific barriers for autistic students, even to a severely disabling degree, if they are overstimulating in terms of noise and other sensory input, while consistency and careful structure of spaces could be an opportunity to ease stress and improve experiences for autistic students. In social and study spaces, students most need the ability to control their environment in terms of distractions, sensory input, and privacy. Campus spaces need to offer students cleanliness, accessibility features, trained and compassionate staff, signage, and feedback mechanisms. All of these issues with campus spaces may be compounded for students with intersecting marginalized identities, such as invisibly disabled and neurodivergent students of color. Finally, dedicated spaces for neurodivergent and disabled students would be helpful, and so would additional supports for managing activities of daily living.

The campus environment can represent a significant source of stress for students, both social and physically. Education and awareness initiatives are a potential approach to improve social environments for students, as are other strategies that will be investigated in Part III. Perhaps the most important takeaway around campus spaces, meanwhile, is that there are two separate categories of need. One is the need to create additional spaces specifically for disabled students, to facilitate their comfort, control, and social connections. Equally important, however, is the need to improve existing spaces, as well as adding new ones. As demonstrated by the difficulty autistic students face with noisy and crowded spaces on campus, while adding accessible spaces is beneficial, it does not make other important parts of campus any more accessible. Making campus a less disabling environment for all students cannot be achieved simply by adding on or repurposing a few individual facilities. Creativity, flexibility, and reorganization will need to be applied to existing classrooms, study spaces, social spaces, and dormitories to make them fully usable by all students. This work is complex and difficult, but if it is not undertaken, distractions, overwhelming sensory input, and other challenges will continue to make multiple parts of campus hostile to some students' needs. The understanding and cooperation of student peers would aid in this work, as would their added advocacy for the needs of their neurodivergent and disabled contemporaries.

6. Intersectional Considerations

As much as this book so far has sought out studies that directly represent students' voices about their own experiences, it is important to note that even the studies I have gathered here do not unproblematically represent all neurodivergent and invisibly disabled students. Of course each study only includes a small sample of students as interviewees, but more importantly, where the demographic distributions of participants are noted, patterns are present that compromise how representative I can claim that this data truly is. In particular, in studies where neurodivergent students were interviewed, participants are frequently described as predominantly white. In fact, a significant number of interview studies with autistic students and those with ADHD had almost entirely or entirely white participants.[1] Neither, of course, is race the only additional marginalized identity that students may have that compounds and changes their experiences of being disabled or neurodivergent in higher education. Unfortunately, however, not all of these intersections are necessarily fully represented or examined in the main body of literature on students' experiences.

This study would be remiss not to examine how students' experiences may vary depending on their other marginalized identities. This chapter will move outside of the main body of literature considered for this book, to include studies of how having other characteristics and identities may alter the experiences of disabled and neurodivergent students. I will discuss how students in my examined categories may be affected by their intersections with race and ethnicity, with gender, and with LGBTQ+ identities. Also to be considered, by way of conclusion, is how trauma may impact students due to their experiences with

---

1   Graves et al., 2011; Randolph, 2012; Schaffer, 2013; Cullen, 2015; Grabsch et al., 2021.

      https://doi.org/10.11647/OBP.0420.06

marginalization, and how all of these intersections may contribute to or mitigate trauma as well.

Intersections with Race and Ethnicity

It is worth noting that, while white participants are generally overrepresented across the majority of studies of higher education experiences, it seems to be mainly around neurodivergent students that this issue is most severe. Studies of student veterans with traumatic brain injuries, psychiatric disabilities, or both tend to be among some of the most racially and ethnically diverse, as do studies of students with traumatic brain injuries in general: Kain et al. (2019) being one example of the former, and Childers and Hux (2016) of the latter. This disproportionality in participants highlights an established and relevant concern: the constructed whiteness of many categories of disability, and in particular of neurodiversity. Kearl (2021) presents a powerful summation of the ways that autism in particular has been socially constructed as a categorization available primarily to white people, while autistic people of color are systematically more likely to be misdiagnosed, diagnosed late, or not diagnosed at all. Clinical studies by Mandell et al. (2002, 2007, 2009) have demonstrated disparities in the age at diagnosis and types of initial misdiagnosis of autism by race, Kearl (2021) notes, while Harry and Klinger (2006) and Losen and Orfield (2002) have helped to identify the racial disparities that occur in placement of students in special education. Black autistic students, in particular, are more likely to be diagnosed with emotional disturbances or intellectual disabilities, because of stereotypical beliefs associating these conditions with Black people, while autism is associated predominantly with whiteness (Losen & Orfield, 2002; Harry & Klinger, 2006). As Kearl (2021) notes, this tendency can be connected to narratives of white innocence and dehumanizing perceptions of Black people in which educators and diagnosticians are unfortunately culturally immersed, which can lead us to classify the same autistic behaviors in white young people as a quirky, harmless, and intellectually-oriented neurodivergence, and in Black young people as violently erratic, threatening, and deficient intellectual conditions and behavioral problems.

Similarly, studies by Morgan et al. (2013, 2014) demonstrate that children of color are less likely to be diagnosed with ADHD or receive medication as treatment than are white children from the ages of nine months through early adolescence; Black children were found to be 69% less likely to be diagnosed, Latino/a/e children 50% less likely, and those from other racial and ethnic groups 46% less likely. While Morgan et al. (2013) speculate that the disparity may partially arise from Black and Latino/a/e parents' reluctance to seek out psychiatric treatment or accept psychiatric diagnoses and medications for their children, which is a reasonable assumption based on prior studies, the similar disparities around diagnosis of autism are also acknowledged. As with autism, another contributing factor may be that what is perceived as a legitimate support need in a white child is at risk of categorization as an inherent behavioral problem in a child of color, and particularly in a Black child due to pervasive anti-Black stereotypes and attitudes. Subsequent studies by Morgan et al. (2015, 2017) have also demonstrated that children with minoritized racial identities are actually less likely than white children to be enrolled in special education or identified as having disability support needs across a wide variety of categorizations, including learning disabilities, speech and language disabilities, health conditions, and emotional disturbances. These observations contradict assumptions that students of color are overrepresented in special education, which have been pervasive for some time. This, too, has likely created well-intentioned hesitancy on the part of educators and parents around the diagnosis of support needs in children of color, for fear of participating in an epidemic of stereotyping pathologization. Parents of children of color in general and of Black children in particular face a troubling double bind when it comes to diagnosing many types of invisible disability: justified fear of negative labeling and misdiagnosis by white-normative educators on one side; consistent patterns of actual underdiagnosis and insufficient support on the other.

Regardless of the reasons for the disparities, one fact remains: neurodivergent and invisibly disabled students of color, particularly Black students, are consistently less likely to be diagnosed prior to or even during higher education. As discussed in previous chapters, this means that they are significantly less likely to be able to access necessary supports and succeed academically, even in comparison to other students with similar needs. It also means that, worse still, less information is available about what their specific needs are. As Crenshaw (1991) noted when elaborating on her originated concept of intersectionality, not only are members of a marginalized community who bear another marginalized identity at risk of having their particular struggles overlooked by that community's advocacy for justice, but the injustices faced by those multiple identities may themselves compound each other.

As Crenshaw also notes, however, 'Intersectional subordination need not be intentionally produced; in fact, it is frequently the consequence of the imposition of one burden that interacts with preexisting vulnerabilities to create yet another dimension of disempowerment' (p. 1249). Likewise, the intersectional subordination of neurodivergent and invisibly disabled students of color that results from their under- or non-representation in these narratives was surely not an intentional omission on the part of researchers—but it is almost certainly a direct consequence of the ways that these students' experiences are impacted by racial and ethnic identities. These students are less likely than their white counterparts to have been correctly diagnosed or diagnosed at all by the time they reach university, meaning they may not be aware of their conditions. Even if they are, they may feel even more alienated from a disability identity than white neurodivergent and invisibly disabled students tend to, given that those types of disabilities in particular are so often rhetorically associated with whiteness. Of course it is reasonable that students of color in these categories would be less likely to put themselves forward as study participants and engage with researchers about their experiences, as a result. Unfortunately, however, this not only means less information is available about serving this student population, but it precludes broader, instructive knowledge of the ways in which neurodivergence and invisible disabilities specifically exacerbate the inequities associated with racial minoritization, and vice versa. Much as it would be preferable to hear from all students in their own voices, and much as we are limited in doing so by whose voices are available, to not address this gap would only perpetuate the existing problems.

To this end, a number of issues deserve particular attention that arise from those studies that do include the narratives of students of color. Cameron and Greenland's (2021) study of two female students of color with dyslexia in the United Kingdom, one south Asian and one Black and multiracial, provides the beginnings of some insight into the compounding issues that may be at work for many students. For example, the authors make specific note of the interviewees' repeated focus on finding 'the right words' to describe their experiences, and how it seemed to be emblematic of their perceived need to live up to exacting expectations in general:

> Lianne: it's interesting that you say 'I'm not putting in the right words' cos you said that a lot in your writing. That you feel like your words are not right. Do you think that you started to feel that you weren't clear when you started your course, or have you always felt like that? Like your words are not right?

> Riya: I've always felt like that to be honest, because, especially when I am in the groups, I'll always end end up saying something I try, I don't want to say, or not not want to say, it just doesn't sound right, and I have to rephrase it, and and, if they, what happened I'd go back by myself and tell myself that I'm stupid? [sort of thing]. (pp. 777-778)

On one side, they felt a sense of hypervisibility, and the need to prove themselves amid the 'model minority' stereotypes and cultural pressures for Asian students in particular, which is also noted in Young's (2012) dissertation on Chinese-American students with ADHD. On the other side, they were likely to experience self-consciousness and stereotype threat around fears of perceived or actual academic inadequacy, especially common for Black students in particular, which is also noted with regard to the Black participants in Childers and Hux's (2016) study of students with mild TBI. The participants in Cameron and Greenland (2021) also describe experiencing university spaces (as opposed to their own personal spaces) as hostile working environments for them, not only because their own personal spaces have affordances that they can use to adapt for their particular learning needs, but also because university spaces are dominated by white men and oriented toward their expectations. Similar experiences are cited by some interviewees in Pfeifer et al. (2021) around participation in STEM programs, where students of color and women already feel pushed out and marginalized by the demographics and assumptions of the field, and find these experiences only exacerbated by the stigma of a learning disability that requires accommodation. Communication and social challenges that neurodivergent and invisibly disabled students may face can also be exacerbated by an accent, cultural differences in word choice and grammatical construction, and other verbal indications of 'otherness' that may be present for English language learners (ELLs) and international students (Cameron & Greenland, 2021). Students from immigrant families in Young (2012) also describe experiences of cultural alienation from their families and community members, not only because of having been raised in a cultural environment other than that of their older family members, but because of their disabilities, and associated stigma and skepticism that may be present in Chinese immigrant communities and others.

There are also a few additional perspectives on the experiences of students of color in these categories, which would otherwise have been scoped out of the literature for examination. Agarwal's (2011) dissertation, for one, examines a study population of mostly Hispanic (Agarwal's choice of term) disabled students at a predominantly Hispanic-serving institution. The interviewees included students with psychiatric disabilities, chronic illness, dyslexia, ADHD, and unspecified learning disability, as well as visual and auditory disabilities and cerebral palsy. It is also notable that the interview participants were on average significantly older than typical undergraduate college age, with all but one interview participant aged twenty-three or older. In students' narratives, however, the barriers they describe facing are very similar to those found in the other studies examined: difficulties with making social connections and relationships, reluctance to request accommodations for fear of stigma, the need to expend significantly more time and effort on academic work than peers, and feeling that disabilities and particularly invisible disabilities are not well understood by faculty. Where identity does seem to play a more significant role for these interviewees, however, is actually in the supports that are available: Agarwal (2011) notes the high importance of family bonds and relationships in Mexican American cultures, which is the cultural context of the vast majority of the participants in this study, and the student narratives extensively credit emotional and practical support from family members for their college success. According to one interviewed student, for example:

> My parents are from Mexico and they are Mexican American. They are family oriented. They provide family support for my education. They support me with transportation. Sometimes when I feel unmotivated, they give me motivation to keep going, also with providing better life, very supportive with whatever I need. . . My parents are my biggest support. I just do the mental aspect of coming to school and take exams. (p. 147)

Especially in light of the recurring value of family support in students' narratives across other studies, the ethnic identity of these students and its associated cultural orientation is clearly an advantage—especially, it seems, when attending a heavily minority-serving institution. Were these students attending a predominantly white institution, it is possible that discrimination and cultural oppression might have imposed more significant barriers.

This assumption seems to be in line with factors observed by Banks (2014) and Booth et al. (2016) in studies of barriers to university transition for young African American men with learning disabilities. Here, stereotype threat magnifies the threat of stigma associated with disclosing disabilities and seeking accommodations. A recurring thread in the young men's narratives is their own, and their families', concerns about race-based negative judgments and stereotypes of their academic abilities if they disclose a need for additional support, leading to shame and embarrassment about help-seeking. Banks (2014) also notes lack of awareness of postsecondary disability services—either that they exist or that they would be available for students with learning disabilities—as a frequent barrier to receiving necessary academic supports. This is especially the case when Black students with invisible disabilities are so likely to have been underidentified and underserved in primary and secondary schooling, including not receiving adequate services for transition to higher education (Banks, 2014). A similar lack was also notably observed in Yamamoto and Black's (2015) study of Native Hawaiian students with learning disabilities facing the transition to higher education, as well as acute feelings of shame and stigma associated with past special education and individualized education plan (IEP) experiences. Similar threads also unite Yamamoto and Black (2015), Booth et al. (2016), and Agarwal (2011) in terms of students' particularly strong family orientations in these studies, with the strongest motivation for postsecondary attendance most often being to support family financially, to live up to family's pride and expectations, or combinations of the two. All of these studies demonstrate and recognize the need to support students in higher education in ways that honor these cultural values and the strengths that they contribute.

Little other information exists on the specific barriers faced by neurodivergent and invisibly disabled undergraduate students of color, with the notable exception of one category: students with psychiatric disabilities. A more robust literature has emerged on racial and ethnic disparities in utilization of college mental health services, which in turn has implications for this category. Certainly, psychiatric disabilities and other mental health struggles are in evidence in students of color, just as in white students, and some evidence suggests students of color may face additional, specific challenges. Kundu (2019) finds that low-income, racially minoritized students are at elevated risk of psychological burnout in college, due to the combination of academic stress with racial battle fatigue and other stressors related to discrimination. In examination of data from the U.S. national Healthy Minds Survey, Lipson et al. (2018) find that Arab American or Arab international students were significantly more likely than other racial demographics to meet criteria for mental health problems, while Han and Pong (2015) note the findings of prior literature that Asian American college students complete suicide at higher rates than those from other racial and ethnic groups, and Canty's (2022) dissertation links mental health challenges for Asian American students at an elite institution to academic stress and impostor syndrome. In spite of these particular concerns, however, students of color have been generally found to underutilize mental health services compared to their white peers, albeit to differing degrees by specific identity. Reasons also vary, but a recurring hypothesis across studies is that cultural norms from families, communities, and countries of origin tend to increase fear and avoidance of stigma for mental health help-seeking.

There is reasonable evidence for this assumption. Miranda et al. (2015) does find that students of color in college counseling were less likely than white students to have been treated previously, less likely to follow through on recommendations, likely to experience worse symptoms, and likely to cite more barriers to treatment, and among these barriers stigma did feature prominently, alongside financial concerns and lack of time. Among other factors, Barksdale and Mollock

(2009) also previously found that negative familial attitudes toward help-seeking had a significant impact on mental health help-seeking for African American students, especially compared against peer attitudes, and especially for women. Masuda et al.'s (2012) study also bears out prior findings that stigma and desire to conceal symptoms were significant factors for African American college students in not seeking out mental health help. Familial and cultural stigma emerge even more strongly as a consideration from an in-depth focus group study by McSpadden (2022) of community college students with predominantly Dominican, Puerto Rican, African American, or African familial origins, or combinations of these. Focus group participants reported negative cultural attitudes in family and home cultures about mental health help-seeking and discussion, as well as frequent preferences for religion or cultural support, fear of racially-bound stigma arising from treatment that might affect life prospects, mistrust of therapy as a practice and associated confidentiality, discomfort with reaching out for help and feeling that it displays weakness, past negative experiences with institutions and staff that decrease trust in counseling services, lack of awareness of services especially as commuters, and discomfort with the idea of mixing treatment with the school setting. Choi and Miller (2014) and Han and Pong (2015) both find, as did prior research, that cultural barriers and stigma are significantly related to the underutilization of mental health services for Asian American and Asian international students, with Choi and Miller (2014) noting that evidence of stronger Asian cultural values was associated with greater stigma avoidance, while greater acculturation to European cultural values was associated with less. Canty (2022) also notes that Asian American students were most likely to attribute their reluctance to seek help to cultural factors in their upbringing.

There is also substantial evidence, however, that the impact of perceived stigma on the help-seeking of students of color is more complex than has been assumed. For example, Cheng et al. (2013) find that African American, Latino American, and Asian American college students perceived varying levels of social stigma around help-seeking, and had internalized that stigma to varying degrees, with greater perceived and internalized stigma corresponding to greater psychological distress and more experiences of racial discrimination. They also find, however, that African American students tended to have lower internalized stigma the stronger their ethnic identity. Similarly, Lipson et al. (2018) find that African American students were likely to perceive the most social stigma around mental health but also have the least internalized stigma. This possibly suggests that strong community bonds and skepticism of the discriminatory attitudes of others may actually buffer the stigma around mental health help-seeking for many African American and Black students, rather than cultural attitudes increasing it. On a similar note, Ramos-Sánchez and Atkinson (2009) find that Mexican American college students were actually more likely to utilize counseling and other mental health services the more enculturated and closer to first-generation they were, which the authors attributed to stronger values in their home culture of interpersonal relationships and support. Among student-athletes, furthermore, the only ethnic group in which Tran (2022) found internalized stigma to correspond to service underutilization was, in fact, white student-athletes. The greater barriers for Black and African American students in various studies tended to center around concern that services would be insufficiently culturally responsive to understand and support their needs (Busby et al., 2021; Samlan et al., 2021), perceptions that their condition was not sufficiently severe to warrant treatment (Busby et al., 2021), lack of time (Busby et al., 2021), and financial concerns (Busby et al., 2021; Samlan et al., 2021). The most significant predictor of help-seeking in Latino/a/e college students in Menendez et al. (2020) was trauma experiences, possibly indicating that help-seeking is seen as a last resort only for cases of severe psychological harm. Perceptions that their symptoms were not sufficiently severe to warrant help-seeking were also more significant than stigma for Asian American students in Kim and Zane (2016), along with greater perceived barriers to treatment and less perceived likely effectiveness than for white students. Gender was also a highly significant factor across multiple ethnic groups in a number of studies, with men less likely to seek treatment than women.[2]

It is apparent that multiple layers of discrimination do affect neurodivergent and invisibly disabled students with other marginalized identities, but of course this is not the only way that students' racial and ethnic identities impact their experiences. Cultural values, community,

---

2   Barksdale & Mollock, 2009; Ramos-Sánchez & Atkinson, 2009; Han & Pong, 2015; Lipson et al., 2018; Tran, 2022.

and identity offer students affordances, support, pride, and comfort that help to bolster them even through specific challenges that may await them in higher education, and possibly more so when they are able to attend institutions that are not predominantly white. It is important to keep in mind that a strong sense of culture and identity is an asset, not a deficit, even when the surrounding culture centers whiteness and marginalized students with other identities. It is as critical to look for ways that students of color can be helped to draw on these supports as it is to eliminate the additional barriers that may be imposed on them.

Intersections with Gender

Overall, there have been some indications that women with disabilities are more likely to graduate from colleges and universities than men (Pingry O'Neill et al., 2012), although gathering precise statistics about higher education students with disabilities is complicated in ways previously discussed. If this is accurate, however, it would also be in line with trends in the general population of college students (National Center for Education Statistics, 2022). Furthermore, a number of other gendered factors may complicate students' experiences, depending on diagnosis and individual symptoms.

As neurodivergence is more likely to be recognized for what it is in white people than in people of color, it is also often more likely to be recognized in men than in women. It is common for neurodivergent young people to display different symptoms and patterns of behavior by gender, often due to associated social pressures and expectations, and diagnosticians are more likely to recognize those presentations that are more common among men. This is particularly true in the case of autistic people, with autistic women more likely to be diagnosed late or not at all (Milner et al., 2019; Cage & Howes, 2020; Krumpelman & Hord, 2021). Several other factors have been suggested as additional explanations for this, including that women may be more motivated to 'fit in' socially (Milner et al., 2019), and specifically seem to be more likely to engage in masking behaviors than men (Lai et al., 2017). A set of strongly gendered stereotypes and expectations are associated with autistic people, as Jack (2014) demonstrates: male 'computer geeks' on one side, emotionally unavailable 'refrigerator mothers' on the other, but with the reality of autistic gender creativity in between. Indeed, discussions of gender and autism are consistently complicated by the relatively frequent occurrence of gender-nonconforming, nonbinary, and transgender identities (or combinations of the three) among autistic people, which has been well documented, and will be discussed further in the next section.

With that said, however, some patterns have been noted of traits that may affect autistic students' experiences by gender, although in most cases the available evidence is limited. There is some evidence of tendencies toward slightly lesser orientation toward patterns and details in autistic women, and toward slightly higher social skills, although these are not unambiguous (Camodeca et al., 2019). There is also some evidence that concurrent mood disorders are most common in autistic women (Kreiser & White, 2015). Socially, autistic women seem to particularly struggle with difficulties in forming and maintaining friendships, and are at greater risk of bullying by peers (Milner et al., 2019; Krumpelman & Hord, 2021). As noted previously, they are also likely to be especially vulnerable in sexual relationships (Milner et al., 2019), and at an even greater risk than other university-aged women of sexual assault (Krumpelman & Hord, 2021). These factors may be related to the fact that, contrary to the general population and disabled students overall, autistic men are actually more likely to persist in college than autistic women, especially if they are enrolled in STEM fields (Wei et al., 2014). Increased likelihood of experiencing emotional disturbances, friendship and relationship difficulties, and sexual assault would certainly make it more difficult for a group of students to finish their degrees.

Similarly to autistic students, there are patterns of characteristics of students with ADHD and dyslexia that vary by gender, and may affect students' experiences. There are some patterns that hold true across both of these categories, as well, although each also has unique patterns. Like autism, both categories are more likely to go unnoticed in women than in men (Hinshaw & Ellison, 2015), likely due to women's having stronger apparent tendencies to develop coping mechanisms, and also to internalize self-blame for their challenges rather than suspecting a disorder (Hoffschmidt & Weinstein, 2003). Hoffschmidt and Weinstein go on to note that these conditions, which they refer to as 'silent learning disorders,' may only surface later in women's lives at major changes of life stage, when suddenly new circumstances render their past coping mechanisms inadequate. Furthermore, there is some evidence that women with ADHD tend to outperform men with ADHD academically (Daffner et al., 2022), and women in both categories appear to demonstrate greater strength in a number of traits potentially impacting academic performance in higher education. For those with ADHD these include fewer memory issues (Kercood et al., 2015) and higher self-determination (Wu & Molina, 2019), and for those with dyslexia they include stronger motivation and time management, and less fear of failure (Tops et al., 2020). University-aged men with ADHD also appear to have more problems than women with 'problematic screen time,' such as excessive gaming impacting academic performance (Hinshaw & Ellison, 2015).

If women in these categories perform better academically, this does impact men more negatively in a number of respects, but it also means that early detection is less likely for women, given that childhood diagnoses tend to result from poor performance in primary and secondary schooling. Otherwise, it is unclear from the existing evidence to what degree, if at all, actual symptoms of these conditions vary by gender. Some studies have found that ADHD appears to cause greater inattention and restlessness issues in women than men (Fedele et al., 2012; Hinshaw & Ellison, 2015; Kercood et al., 2015), but Schepman et al. (2012) finds the opposite to be true. Fedele et al. (2012) also find women with ADHD to have greater impairment across most areas of daily life, but this was derived from a self-report study with minimal corroborating data available, which the authors acknowledge as a limitation—and which may mean that women with ADHD are simply more likely to negatively evaluate their own life skills.

Indeed, it is socially and emotionally where the most pronounced complications appear to exist specifically for women in both categories. Women who already feel marginalized in male-dominated fields like STEM then feel even more undermined by identifying with a condition like ADHD or dyslexia (Pfeifer et al., 2021), and these impacts are compounded even further for women of color (Cameron & Greenland, 2021). Women's romantic relationships appear to be more negatively impacted by ADHD symptoms, especially when those symptoms are more severe (Bruner et al., 2015), and adolescent girls and young women with ADHD are more likely than others to experience relationship violence (Hinshaw & Ellison, 2015). In terms of mental health, ADHD medications are associated with a risk of eating disorder misuse, of which university-aged women are particularly at risk (Gibbs et al., 2016). As with autism, co-occurrence of depression and anxiety with dyslexia is more common in women (Nelson & Gregg, 2012). Negative emotional experiences appear to be more common in women both with and without ADHD than men, although all university-aged people with ADHD appear to have more negative emotional experiences than those without (Kearns & Ruebel, 2011). Women with ADHD are also at elevated risk of suicide and self-harm, and are more likely than men to have experienced trauma in early life, such as childhood abuse (Hinshaw & Ellison, 2015).

Among students with TBI, as well, social and emotional challenges in particular also seem to be more common for women than for men (Mukherjee et al., 2003). All of these patterns, even across other categories, align with data indicating that psychiatric disabilities are more commonly diagnosed in women than in men (National Institute of Mental Health, 2023a), especially eating disorders (National Institute of Mental Health, 2023b). When considering these data, however, it is worth keeping in mind that women are historically more likely to be psychiatrically pathologized for both benign personality differences and physical ailments (Poulin & Gouliquer, 2003). These patterns may also impact some women more than others, or impacts may vary. In the U.S., in particular, white women are more likely to be diagnosed with a psychiatric illness as the result of trauma than are women of any other race or ethnicity who have experienced trauma (Townsend et al., 2020). This could be the result of a buffer effect from ethnic identity, as Townsend suggests, or it may be that women of color are perceived as less vulnerable and therefore underdiagnosed, or a combination of these and other factors. In any case, overall, university-aged women are also more likely to experience significant mental health impacts from trauma history involving sexual assault (Zinzow et al., 2011), and women with common conditions like depression report similar patterns of significant impact on their studies from their symptoms, including in online learning (Orr, 2021). Other marginalized identities, such as race and ethnicity or LGBTQ+ identities, may also compound women's risk factors, as not only major trauma associated with marginalization but even more minor and repeated forms of harm like microaggressions have demonstrable mental health impacts (Boyle et al., 2022).

Interestingly, and perhaps relatedly, one study of college students found evidence of lower self-compassion among students with mental health symptoms and in mental health treatment, and also independently among women (Lockard et al., 2014). Some similar factors may affect both groups, but it is also likely that there is significant overlap between the two, given women's greater diagnosis rates and also their apparent higher likelihood of seeking help for mental health concerns. For example, while women appear to have higher rates of psychological distress than men among student athletes (Sullivan et al., 2019), they also report being more willing to seek help than do men, with no difference between athletes and non-athletes (Barnard, 2016). Masculinity and gender norms appear to be major factors in preventing men from seeking help with mental health issues, and, as noted in the earlier section on race and ethnicity, there is a pervasive pattern of men being relatively unwilling to seek treatment (Assadi, 2021). This is concerning for multiple reasons, but partly because untreated mental health symptoms in men may be more likely than those in women to translate into harm to those around them: for example, symptoms of social anxiety have been linked to an increased risk of attempting sexual assault or other forms of sexual aggression in undergraduate university-aged men (Calzada et al., 2011).

Chronic illness, meanwhile, may not affect women more frequently than men, but it may impact them in particular ways. Chronic pain conditions, for example, have been found to be more common in those with a history of childhood or domestic abuse, of which women are more likely to be survivors (Kendall-Tackett et al., 2003). Struggling to be diagnosed or even believed, whether by peers or by medical professionals, is a common experience among those with chronic invisible conditions, and this is especially true for women, making it more likely they will be hampered in receiving treatment and support (Moss & Dyck, 2003). Certain conditions are also especially gendered, especially stigmatized, or both: for example, myalgic encephalomyelitis (ME), often called chronic fatigue syndrome, is both significantly more prevalent in women and treated with significant skepticism even by medical practitioners (Moss & Dyck, 2003). There are significantly higher expectations of domestic work and emotional caretaking from women in heterosexual romantic relationships than of men, which may impact women's relationships if their health limits their perceived ability to meet those expectations; this may impact university-aged women less than those later in life, but situations vary (Moss & Dyck, 2003). In any case, as in all categories, differences in social expectations and probable life experiences by gender have a major impact on how strongly and in what ways chronic illness affects students.

Intersections with LGBTQ+ Identities

Not only do LGBTQ+ identities significantly overlap with neurodivergence and invisible disabilities, but the considerations of both identities parallel and interact with one another in a number of ways. While Samuels (2003) has rightly cautioned against simplistically conflating the experiences of LGBTQ+ and disabled people, and emphasizes the need to remain mindful of the complexities and nuances of each, there are patterns of LGBTQ+ student experience that will be very familiar after having detailed those of invisibly disabled and neurodivergent students. As with gender, scholars have begun increasingly to place queer theory and disability theory in conversation with one another, bringing an additional lens of analysis to both. Kafer's (2013) *Feminist, Queer, Crip*, for example, argues for the intertwined nature of compulsory heterosexuality and compulsory able-bodiedness as cultural forces, and Walker's (2021) *Neuroqueer Heresies* details the author's bringing the concept of 'queering' discourse into the development of the neurodiversity paradigm. Walker's radical rhetorical expansion of possibilities for neurobiological functioning is fundamentally linked with similar expansions of possibilities for sexuality and gender, and it offers a means of simultaneous and intertwined resistance to both neuro- and heteronormativity.

For our purposes, however, of most interest are the ways that lived experiences of LGBTQ+ identity, neurodivergence, and invisible disabilities interact with each other for students. Perhaps most notably, both types of identities share the commonality that they are invisible unless students choose to disclose them. One of the most commonly mentioned areas of overlap is that in both cases, many students work to consciously manage others' perceptions of themselves, and carefully choose whether, when, and how to disclose information about their identities, because of the risk of stigma and discrimination.[3] Students describe the invisibility of their identities as a 'double-edged sword,' protecting them to a degree from stigma but also obstructing their positive self-identification (Miller et al., 2019), which leads to experiences of what one student describes as being 'closeted twice' (Miller, 2018, p. 337). Depending on context, students may feel the need to pass as those with more privileged identities in multiple dimensions, to manage risk and protect themselves (Miller et al., 2019; Abrams & Abes, 2021).

Even beyond the issue of visibility, as well, the LGBTQ+ experiences of students in both identity groups present curious echoes of recurring themes in invisibly disabled and neurodivergent students' narratives. For example, as disabled students are expected to advocate for their needs to faculty and risk exposure and stigma in the process, the onus to challenge heterosexism, homophobia, and transphobia in the classroom, curriculum, or college environment often falls on LGBTQ+ students, rather than being addressed at the institutional level, but to do so risks unwanted personal exposure (Daniels & Geiger, 2010; Miller, 2015; Bell, 2017). LGBTQ+ students, especially those who are disabled and neurodivergent, are often on an additional cultural learning curve when it comes to adapting to the university environment, creating time disadvantages not unlike those experienced by disabled students generally (Daniels & Geiger, 2010). In fact, Daniels and Geiger (2010) go so far as to propose modifying and repurposing the Universal Design for Learning framework, designed for inclusion of disabled students, as a tool for the inclusion of LGBTQ+ students as well, recognizing the similarities and overlap between the two groups.

Furthermore, the stigma and discrimination faced by each group tend not only to coincide with, but to be compounded by their combination (Miller, 2015; Bell, 2017). For example, the infantilization and desexualization to which disabled people are frequently subject tends to play into dismissals of LGBTQ+ identity as 'just a phase' or 'confusion' (Toft et al., 2019). A recent study, comparing LGBQ+ students

---

3   Daniels & Geiger, 2010; Miller, 2015; Bell, 2017; Miller et al., 2017; Miller, 2018; Miller et al., 2019; Toft et al., 2019; Miller & Smith, 2021.

specifically and disabled students against their peers with respectively more privileged identities, also found that the LGBQ+ group and the disabled group was each significantly more likely to have more negative experiences, such as feeling physically unsafe, not being able to be themselves, not feeling they belonged, and being discriminated against (BrckaLorenz et al., 2020). These negative experiences were significantly higher than for either of those single identity groups for students who identified as both LGBQ+ and disabled. Other studies have also found that some of the discrimination experienced by transgender and gender-nonconforming disabled students parallel those of disabled cisgender women students, creating a useful grouping of disabled 'gender minorities'; the intersections of both sets of identities led to perceptions of weakness and inability by the students who shared them, and increased those students' feelings of being unsafe and at risk of violence (Kimball et al., 2018; Vaccaro et al., 2020).

Another negative commonality of LGBTQ+ and disabled identities is that students regularly experience microaggressions from higher education faculty and staff about both types of identity (Bell, 2017). Several student narratives also describe experiences of family or higher education employees falsely conflating their LGBTQ+ identity with their disability or neurodivergence, or incorrectly assigning responsibility for one identity to the other, to students' frustration (Bell, 2017; Toft et al., 2019). More common types of microaggression from a broader study, however, appear to be denial or minimization of either or both identities, imposing heteronormative and gender normative expectations, misgendering, treating disability as an imposition, structural inaccessibility of spaces and activities to students because of one or both identities, and racist or other intersectional microaggressions, including in white-dominated LGBTQ+ and/or disability-friendly spaces (Miller & Smith, 2021). As the same study points out, all of these types of discrimination are insidiously vague and difficult to pinpoint, although they significantly and negatively impact students' lives. Students with both identities may also be poorly positioned to confront discrimination against one identity because of the impacts of the other: for example, an autistic or psychiatrically disabled student may feel intense discomfort confronting someone else socially for a homophobic remark, or a gender-nonconforming student may find they are not taken seriously about their disability needs because of stigma around their gender presentation (Miller & Smith, 2021). Furthermore, both identities are also similar in their frequent invisibility or stigmatization within the curriculum. As one student notes even of a course with intentionally diverse assigned readings, 'We don't get a gay book,' and the same can often be said for representation of disabled voices (Miller, 2015, p. 388).

Gender identity, in particular, represents another site of potential difficulty that may intersect with neurodivergence and disability. Recognizing and embracing one's identity as transgender, nonbinary, or otherwise gender-nonconforming can be an emotional and demanding journey for anyone at a university student's stage of life, and doubly so for a student already burdened by additional pressures around being invisibly disabled or neurodivergent (Kimball et al., 2018; Cain & Velasco, 2021). Effective and consistent medical transition care can also be extremely hard to obtain, especially in some geographical areas and for students with higher body weights, and can present challenging interactions with other medical conditions (Cain & Velasco, 2021). There is a critical need for specifically trans-aware mental health and medical support on college campuses, and one that, as has already been demonstrated, is not always well met (Cain & Velasco, 2021). Even students who are willing to overcome the obstacles to their appropriate gender-affirming care may still be hesitant, because of fears of how they may be perceived and stigmatized by others (Kimball et al., 2018; Cain & Velasco, 2021). Neither are these fears unfounded, especially for disabled students. Disabled transgender students are at demonstrably greater risk than even disabled LGBQ+ students of direct microaggressions and victimization (Miller et al., 2021), and are more likely to experience significant discrimination, harassment, violence, and economic precarity. As a direct result of this last factor, a significant percentage of disabled transgender college students will at some point engage in sex work, for which they seldom have access to sufficient health and safety resources on campus (Coston et al., 2022).

On the whole, invisibly disabled and neurodivergent students who are also LGBTQ+ are consistently likely to face significantly greater hardships than their non-LGBTQ+ peers, who face significant hardships compared to neurotypical and nondisabled students already. The impacts of these experiences also have implications for how factors like positive disability identity help to support student success. As several narrative studies have shown, rather than being able to have an organic 'identity development' experience as LGBTQ+ or disabled, these students find their identities forcibly shaped and made to shift by discrimination and oppressive environments (Kimball et al., 2018; Abrams & Abes, 2021). Because their marginalized identities are invisible, in particular, students are frequently forced into being perceived through a lens of compulsory heterosexuality and able-bodiedness, making it more difficult to have their needs recognized and supported (Kimball et al., 2018; Abrams & Abes, 2021). It is worthwhile to note, however, that whiteness and physical features still mitigate these impacts, and racial and ethnic marginalization as well as appearance factors, such as body size or obvious disfiguration, compound them (Abrams & Abes, 2021).

Even as these identities develop in whatever form they are able, they may also come into conflict with each other. Students may feel uncomfortable and ill-suited to LGBTQ+ spaces due to their disabilities or neurodivergence, such as when LGBTQ+ gatherings are sensorily or socially prohibitive for autistic students or trigger anxiety in psychiatrically disabled students, or they may feel their LGBTQ+ identity is not accepted in spaces and gatherings for disabled students (Miller et al., 2017; Miller, 2018). For example, one student described his experience with LGBTQ+ spaces on campus:

> I went into the gay youth help thingy center and it was political. It had sort of that angry atmosphere that I just . . . and it was cliquish and so I just thought about going to some of the meetings that they have, but I mean I have anxiety problems and going to something like that alone: that's not great. (Miller et al., 2017, p. 128)

Some students may embrace their LGBTQ+ identity but feel the need to distance themselves from a disabled one (Bell, 2017; Miller et al., 2017; Miller, 2018; Toft et al., 2019), or the other way around (Miller et al., 2017), depending on the student's individual experiences and concerns. Still other students, however, see the two identities as integrated and in conversation with each other; this is especially common in studies with participant groups that skew older, such as mixed undergraduate and graduate student studies, and may be a conclusion at which students increasingly arrive over time (Miller, 2018). Considering the two to be intertwined appears to be especially likely for transgender and otherwise gender-nonconforming autistic students,[4] and for LGBTQ+ students with psychiatric disabilities, particularly anxiety and depression (Miller, 2018). There also seem to be some patterns of co-occurrence that support these impressions. It has been established in the literature that autistic people are substantially more likely than others to be transgender, gender-nonconforming, or otherwise LGBTQ+ (de Vries et al., 2010; Shmulsky & Gobbo, 2019), and there is in fact some evidence of correlation between autism and intersex traits at the biological level (Bejerot et al., 2012). A study of only LGBQ+ disabled students, meanwhile, found mental illness to be the most commonly occurring disability among them (BrckaLorenz et al., 2020), and depression is also a frequently reported factor negatively impacting well-being in LGBTQ+ disabled students (Miller et al., 2021). As with other ways that LGBTQ+ students are underserved, however, treatment for these disabilities seems to be less common even as their occurrence is proportionally higher. LGBTQ+ students with anxiety and depression have been found to be less likely than others to be in treatment, except at high levels of severity of symptoms (Seehuus et al., 2021), and veterans with minoritized sexual orientations have been found to be significantly more likely both to have post-traumatic stress disorder (PTSD) and to have military sexual trauma exposure, but significantly less likely to be receiving services for these as disabilities (Shipherd et al., 2021).

More encouragingly, however, links between the two identities have also been established as positive influences on student well-being. LGBTQ+ pride and strong peer support networks have both been found to support well-being for these students (Miller et al., 2021). Furthermore, when students do choose to disclose one or both of their identities, a commonly recurring reason for doing so is to show solidarity and support for others (Miller et al., 2019). When students feel particularly isolated and excluded based on their identities, especially in disciplines like STEM that tend to have more heteronormative, inaccessible, and unsupportive cultures, in many cases they choose to respond by increasing their personal visibility as a representative of marginalized identities, and advocating for change (Miller & Downey, 2020). Abrams and Abes (2021) and their interviewee characterize this

---

4   Miller et al., 2017; Kimball et al., 2018; Toft et al., 2019; Cain & Velasco, 2021.

type of resistance as 'radical self-love,' and describe the positive impacts for the student of rejecting traditional structures and expectations, and advocating against injustice in spite of the discomfort of visibility and negative perceptions (Abrams & Abes, 2021). As difficult as it can be for students to claim their identities and be visible, and as much as it would be better to be in positive environments where they do not need to advocate to be seen and supported, engaging in these activities can nonetheless serve as one path for students to develop a sense of positive identity that helps to sustain them.

Intersections with Trauma

Some degree of trauma history is common for students with marginalized identities, including disabled students, and the risk is increased for every additional marginalized identity a student has. Increased likelihood of exposure to trauma and posttraumatic symptoms have been linked to race and ethnicity (A.L. Roberts et al., 2011), disability (Harrell, 2017; Liasidou, 2023), sexual and gender minoritization (Coulter & Rankin, 2020), and intersections of all of these (Seng et al., 2012). College students with ADHD since childhood, in particular, have been found to be significantly more likely to have a trauma exposure history and/or PTSD symptoms (Miodus et al., 2021). It is therefore vital, as we consider the ways in which intersecting identities are likely to impact students' experiences, to also consider the ways that students are impacted by trauma.

A personal history of trauma, whether or not the person who experienced it has developed PTSD or not, has multiple significant effects on day-to-day life, especially for college students. Because of the way memory is processed during an extremely stressful or dangerous event, later in life the person who experienced the trauma may have a fight, flight, or freeze response even during nonthreatening events or situations, may relive or reexperience part or all of the initial traumatic event, and may develop coping behaviors like disassociation, hypervigilance, or avoidance, along with numerous other possible changes to mood, cognition, behavior, and sleep (Conley et al., 2019). For students in higher education in particular, there is evidence that a history of trauma significantly impacts academic performance and overall quality of life (Goodman, 2017). This is particularly concerning given that, as we have seen, disabled students are already often at a significant disadvantage in these areas, which the addition of trauma symptoms may well make seemingly insurmountable. In many very real ways, trauma is itself disabling, whether or not the psychological impacts from trauma constitute the student's primary disability. As Liasidou (2023) articulates, trauma and disability are not one another, but they are deeply interrelated, and impact and arise from one another. Furthermore, particularly for marginalized students including disabled students, and especially for multiply marginalized students, higher education itself can be a traumatic experience:

> I'd got myself into such a state about it, and then I just ended up having some sort of meltdown over it. And I think just the stress of it had been building and it's such an intense feeling. The kind of response is to just run away and go well I just don't want to feel like that again. So, I thought I just can't do it [the degree]. (Cage & Howes, 2020, p. 1669)

Even students who begin higher education neurodivergent or invisibly disabled but with no trauma history may not remain without one for long, in the face of peer and faculty stigma and discrimination, insufficient support, and systems that set them up to fail at every turn.

To help mitigate the additional impacts of trauma on students already operating under multiple other burdens, higher education faculty, staff, and administrators may consider a variety of strategies. Being aware of the risk of microaggressions and working proactively to prevent them, gently disrupting students' negative self-talk in support interactions, providing self-service mental health support resources that students can access anonymously and discreetly, developing programming in support of marginalized identities especially with leadership representative of those identities, working to increase staff and faculty diversity, and carefully referring students to appropriate services on campus as need arises have all been suggested as small steps that could be taken to improve the experiences of students with trauma histories (Conley et al., 2019). The availability of robust counseling and other mental health services on campus is also a critical imperative (Goodman, 2017). To faculty in particular, Orem and Simpkins (2015) strongly recommend a thoughtful implementation of the practice of trigger warnings for course content. Rather than avoiding making students engage with any uncomfortable topics, they argue, these warnings deliberately share control of students' experiences in class with the students themselves, providing students the means of recognizing and managing their own mental health needs and allowing them to engage with difficult and sensitive material on their own terms, without being harmed or excluded.

Summary and Conclusions

Neurodivergent and invisibly disabled students are already marginalized based on these identities, but they may also have other marginalized identities that intersect and interact with these in a number of ways. Neurodivergent students of all other races, ethnicities, and genders are less likely than white male students to have their needs recognized and supported appropriately. Students of color, non-male students, LGBTQ+ students, and all combinations thereof may feel excluded and isolated in campus spaces due to those identities, particularly in certain disciplines where privileged identities tend to dominate, and being disabled or neurodivergent only compounds that experience. With each type of intersecting identity, however, the ways that they interact are not simple, and not necessarily negative. Stereotype threat and cultural attitudes may particularly deter accessing supports for students of color, particularly those with psychiatric disabilities—but at the same time, strong racial and ethnic identities and cultural factors can be emotional supports and motivators that increase student success and help-seeking. Women are generally more vulnerable to abuse, violence, and social or emotional challenges, and tend to have lower estimations of their own abilities and less self-compassion, but they are also more likely than men with similar conditions to succeed academically, to seek and receive support, and to express symptoms in ways that do not bring harm to others. Invisible disabilities and LGBTQ+ identities impact students in curiously similar and intertwined ways, and students with either identity experience more negative impacts on their quality of life than students with privileged identities, while students with both experience the most negative impacts of all. They struggle with invisibility and erasure, stigma and discrimination that are sometimes violent, medical and emotional challenges around gender identity and transition, and a climate that is generally hostile to their formation of a positive identity. Their identities may also come into conflict with one another in ways that prevent their receiving full needed support. And yet, many see those identities as deeply interrelated and formative, and claiming and advocating for them can be a source of pride, strength, and community that is sustaining.

Across many studies, students report experiences of being excluded and made to suffer for their marginalized identities, but those identities can also just as often be a valuable and nourishing part of their lives. It is important to recognize and celebrate these critical parts of who students are, and at the same time, to be mindful of the increased likelihood that they have been harmed in ways that will continue to impact them in higher education. Disabled and neurodivergent students are more likely than others to have experienced trauma, and more so with each additional marginalized identity they may have, which has significant and often additionally disabling psychological impacts that affect their success and their quality of life. Inclusive faculty and staff must work to increase their awareness of the needs these factors create, and employ additional strategies to meet them. If we seek to support neurodivergent and invisibly disabled students, we must be committed to supporting all of them, from those who have been at the greatest disadvantage from the combination of factors affecting their lives to those who have been at the least. Inclusive support that is mindful of the intersecting impacts of marginalization, and of trauma, will benefit all students, but it will most benefit those who are most in need.

PART III

DIRECTIONS FOR POSITIVE CHANGE

7. Curricular Support Strategies

Because much of the purpose of investigating students' experiences is to uncover barriers, this book so far may feel like simply a long list of problems. It is important to recognize that the issues these students face in higher education are numerous, and to the serious detriment of their educational experiences. This should not imply, however, that these problems are without solutions, or that educational institutions have made no attempts to date to address them. On the contrary, both students' narratives and other areas of the literature reveal promising practices that could be or have been implemented already. In some areas these practices are still emerging, and have yet to achieve their full potential, but even experimental attempts provide valuable ideas for paths forward.

This chapter will review examples of practices that students have suggested would be helpful, and strategies institutions have tried to meet their needs. These fall into four general categories, emerging from common themes across student narratives:

1. Needs for structural change at the university level that students may not have explicitly identified, but that are implicit in their experiences;

2. Proactive outreach and intervention by disability services and others;

3. Assistive technologies provided by the institution; and

4. Mentoring services from peers and others in the college or university.

While these are clear needs for a majority of students, the degree to which they have been addressed at educational institutions varies widely. Examples of some are nearly nonexistent in the literature, and

©2024 Ash Lierman, CC BY-NC 4.0   https://doi.org/10.11647/OBP.0420.07

others are well-established and -documented areas of practice. It should come as no surprise that the least progress has been made toward many of the more fundamental, structural changes, while substantial work has been done on simpler and less far-reaching interventions. Nonetheless, even small changes can have a significant impact for a struggling community, and even the most modest program that shows promise should be considered.

Implicit and Structural Needs

Time Flexibility and Beyond

There is scarcely any need to repeat the significance of the outsized time and effort demands placed upon invisibly disabled and neurodivergent students. This has been one of the most pervasive and critical themes observed throughout this work. How to address this issue, however, is a more complicated question, and one for which educational institutions have neither found a clear answer nor even, it seems, made significant progress in searching for one. If some students need more time than others, in order to complete their academic work and also to manage other time-consuming aspects of their lives, what can institutions reasonably do to give it to them?

In theory, flexible approaches to learning time would seem to be a potential solution, and one in line with the principles of Universal Design for Learning (UDL). For those unfamiliar, UDL is a framework for accessibility in education developed by the Center for Applied Special Technology (CAST). It derives from the Universal Design (UD) framework in architecture, which promotes collaborating with disabled people in architectural design processes to create buildings with access for all considered in their fundamental structure, rather than requiring cumbersome and ineffectual retrofits to compensate for accessibility barriers. UDL applies similar principles to education, encouraging educational designs that take difference into account from the beginning, provide flexibility and multiple pathways for learners, and recognize that the mechanics of instruction can and should be altered according to what will best facilitate learning for individuals. While UDL has seen more significant adoption in primary and secondary education, where stricter legislation governs the inclusion of disabled students, it has begun to make inroads in higher education as well: Tobin and Behling (2018), for example, have contributed one prominent guide to practical application. Although CAST's guidelines for UDL recommend multiple aspects of flexibility (CAST, 2018), however, they do not mention altering the *time* that learners receive to process material and demonstrate their knowledge. Some educators may interpret leniency around time as an aspect of applied UDL, but the CAST guidelines do not explicitly call for it.

Of course, this may be for the very practical reason of keeping the guidelines from seeming impossible to implement. Primary, secondary, and higher education proceed on extremely regimented schedules in their own ways, which individual instructors have little ability to influence. Academic years, semesters, and quarters are set at the administrative level of the institution or even higher, at the level of local government, and for myriad reasons are not subject to change. Suggesting that students should be able to learn at their own pace, within these systems, would be more likely to result in educators rejecting the UDL framework outright as unfeasible, rather than any transformative change to their practice. This is also most likely partly why so little work has been done on investigating these types of approaches, in higher education or beyond.

With that said, within the literature around higher education, there have been some modest attempts to implement time flexibility in teaching, although these have generally been made by individual instructors within the confines of individual courses. A number of authors describe practicing and advocating flexible course deadlines with no penalties for late work, as a means of creating a caring campus environment and encouraging students' sense of belonging, largely in response to the COVID-19 pandemic (Kruger et al., 2022; Barnett & Cho, 2023; Kruger, 2023; Robinson et al., 2023), and sometimes in recognition of the same time inequities for disabled and neurodivergent students as have been noted here (Hills & Peacock, 2022). Other studies implementing similar strategies in courses have documented positive impacts of these on students' course success (Withington & Schroeder, 2017; Miller et al., 2019). Although these changes may be relatively small, they represent a positive step, and it is also likely that far more faculty use similar practices than have published studies of them.

There is also at least one slightly more radical experiment to be noted: the FreeStartFreePace program at Dalarna University in Falun, Sweden, which authors describe as an example of 'flexible study pace' (Wissa & Avdic, 2017). This was an e-learning program that allowed students significantly more freedom than is traditional in when to start and complete courses, and was specifically implemented as a UDL-based, disability-oriented intervention. The authors reported some positive affective responses from students to the program, but also mixed results in terms of academic success—which may be at least as related to its online mode as to other factors, given students' variable success rates with online and face-to-face learning as noted in Chapter 4. It is difficult to say at the present moment how or if this structure could function in a face-to-face setting, for that matter. Even so, with care for the structure of the online learning environment, a time-flexible online alternative to time-rigid face-to-face instruction could be a better option than none at all. As this program was designed to accord with UDL principles, it can also serve as an example of Tobin & Behling's (2018) 'plus-one approach': working to ease just one common sticking point for students at a time, in recognition that improving learning design is an ongoing, iterative process (p. 134). Creating additional alternatives is often more valuable as well as more feasible than perfecting the accessibility of an entire course or program.

There might be more promise to report from this example, however, if the FreeStartFreePace program were still in place to this day, but from investigation of Dalarna University's current program information, it does not appear to be. Neither does any evidence seem to exist that any other institution has tried a similar approach since 2017. The challenges of the COVID-19 pandemic era may have deterred innovation in this area, at least temporarily, as has also seemed to be the cause of many Western institutions' waning interest in hosting massively open online courses (MOOCs), although these do continue to flourish in other parts of the world (Tlili et al., 2022). While individual instructors may explore time flexibility in individual courses, the standard academic term seems to remain overwhelmingly non-negotiable overall, and this still leaves students' time at the mercy of circumstance and which faculty members they are lucky (or unlucky) enough to encounter. It is also unfortunate that this lack of imagination around academic terms exists when it comes to students who need more time, as the same is not true for students who want to spend *less* time: standard academic terms have certainly proven to be mutable before, but in the form of accelerated and block-plan schedules, for example, and not relaxed or extended schedules.

There are, however, legitimate reasons that extending students' time in college might not be desirable or beneficial. Students have a number of financial and personal pressures to finish college faster than not, including the costs that accumulate from college attendance and the delay of better employment opportunities available with a degree (Urban Institute, n.d.). At the very least, the financial burdens of university would need to be allayed before true time flexibility would be feasible from a student's perspective, at least in the U.S. and other nations where higher education is so costly. From an institutional perspective, meanwhile, there are additional incentives to graduate students within a traditional time frame, as in many cases official graduation rates for an institution are only calculated from student completion within these time frames. Even beyond this factor, evidence also suggests that taking longer to complete college reduces academic momentum, ultimately leading to a higher likelihood of attrition before graduating (Conway et al., 2021). This only decreases the attractiveness of allowing students more time in their academic programs, for both students and academic institutions.

At the same time, time struggles are real and severe for invisibly disabled and neurodivergent students as well as for other marginalized communities, negatively impacting both their academic work and their quality of life. Individual faculty members' efforts in individual courses to ameliorate them are a positive step and beneficial, but can only extend so far: faculty are also beholden to university schedules in ways that constrain how much flexibility they are really able to provide, and their workloads and course structure may suffer for trying to be more accommodating than a restrictive institutional-level calendar will allow. As many teaching faculty know intimately, even providing deadline extensions within a course can cause new stressors and bottlenecks of work for both the instructor and the student (Hewett et al., 2017). When only some faculty are attempting to provide flexibility, more flexible courses may end up with reduced engagement in favor of those less flexible: for example, high-demand times in their other courses have been shown to be a cause of increased student absenteeism in class (Oldfield et al., 2018). Tobin and Behling (2018) also affirm that UDL cannot be fully achieved alone, and broad implementation of the framework is needed in order to make significant change (p. 145). Indeed, a potential remedy to the stated problems of providing only individual, constrained pockets of flexibility may lie in their tenth chapter, on creating a culture of UDL campus-wide. An entire institutional environment where staff and faculty have embraced the need to coordinate efforts to reduce students' time pressures could be tremendously beneficial—although no examples of such an environment seem to exist just yet. The example in Tobin and Behling (2018) of the University of South Dakota's cultural shift, however, demonstrates that it is possible to move an entire campus together toward widespread adoption of UDL principles. Could the principle of time flexibility not be added to them?

The concept of time poverty could provide a common language and framing for approaching such efforts. Giurge et al. (2020) put forward the notion of time poverty as an increasingly prevalent deficit of the time individuals have available relative to their responsibilities, which they find to be linked to poorer well-being, health, and productivity, even though being short of time may be socially normalized and even valorized. While these impacts occur on the individual level, furthermore, they note that time poverty results from numerous societal and systemic shifts beyond individuals' control, and in many cases may be linked to financial and material poverty. Time poverty is an emerging concept in the social sciences, and at an early stage of study; consequently, little data is available so far on its impacts across other strata of marginalization. Giurge et al. (2020), however, theorize that time poverty is likely to be more common within marginalized communities, and point to a need for more study and data collection in this area. Whillans and West (2022) continued this work by investigating time poverty and its impacts among the working poor, and found that any increase in available material resources, whether time-focused or not, helped to alleviate its impacts. They also identified pathways by which material poverty becomes a direct cause of time poverty: such as the fact that study participants universally reported choosing to sacrifice time in favor of money (for example, never paying for time-saving services).

The demonstrated disadvantages neurodivergent and invisibly disabled students face, both in time and financial resources, should be sufficient to identify them as a time-impoverished population. Neither are they alone among college students, as recent early explorations into time poverty in higher education have shown. Most recently, time poverty has been found to be a factor in different educational outcomes by race and gender (Wladis et al., 2024), and student parents have also been identified as disproportionately time-impoverished compared to other students, with impacts also significantly varying by gender (Conway et al., 2021). In both cases, as with disabled and neurodivergent students, time poverty leads the population in question to expend a higher proportion of time on academic study rather than other aspects of life compared with other populations, often sacrificing time spent on activities needed for overall well-being. These effects are likely only compounded for crossovers of these groups, and by additional marginalized identities that individuals in any one group may hold. Gray (2021) even goes so far as to identify all writing students as a time-impoverished population, and investigates the intervention of a 'slow writing' instructional pace that would seek to reduce the pace of writing-intensive courses to improve outcomes—an approach that overlaps with the above discussion of time flexibility.

Conway et al. (2021), however, propose a bolder solution that may be more in line with the broader research on time poverty: including the alleviation of time poverty as a factor in financial aid decisions, along with increasing other campus resources that can relieve time and other forms of poverty. These may include campus interventions for food and housing insecurity, funding for materials and technologies needed for study, provision of child and other dependent care, and more. While, to the best of my knowledge, factoring time hardship alongside financial hardship in determining need for aid is a purely theoretical concept at this point, it is one that holds the potential to address time poverty in the ways that the research to date has indicated may be most beneficial. As Whillans and West's (2022) findings have suggested, having more financial resources in general would help address students' time poverty in a variety of ways: it would reduce the need to add outside employment to students' already overloaded schedules, enable access to time-saving services and technologies, and reduce the stress and mental health pressures of precarity. It would also best serve a wide variety of student populations who disproportionately experience time poverty, well beyond invisibly disabled and neurodivergent students— as opposed to other, more gatekeeping possibilities, such as providing time-saving services as an accommodation for demonstrated disability. Indeed, the requirement to prove disability in order to qualify for accommodations is already a problematic and significant burden that it is similarly important to address.

Accommodations Documentation

In *Academic Ableism*, Dolmage (2018) clearly articulates the problem with required documentation for accommodations: it places the onus upon students to prove that they 'deserve' provisions to which they are in fact legally entitled under the ADA, and in effect presents a new barrier more than it enables access. Dolmage continues:

> There is a clear rhetoric in this accommodation discourse as well, an attitude of indifference toward the individual, and a refusal to provide support until this support is legally mandated. Following this process, the accommodations offered still demand that the student must accommodate him or herself to the dominant logic of classroom pedagogy. Once we begin to go down the road of accommodating disability, we are also admitting that dominant pedagogies privilege those who can most easily ignore their bodies, and those whose minds work the most like the minds of their teachers (likely meaning, as well, those who look much like their teachers). (p. 80)

Movement away from the accommodations-by-request model remains almost nonexistent in higher education, in spite of the inequities that Dolmage and other have shown it to exacerbate. Even movement away from onerous requirements for documentation has begun to occur only modestly. One critical development in this area has been the 2012 guidelines from the Association on Higher Education and Disability (AHEAD), which emphasize 'non-burdensome process' for students to obtain accommodations, underscore students' legal entitlement to a higher education that accommodates their disabilities, and, most importantly, recommend student self-report as the primary form of documentation for making accommodations decisions (AHEAD, 2012). While this was a promising development in 2012, from the literature it appears to have been incorporated into actual disability services practice only gradually over the past decade. In recent years, however, disability services professionals have increasingly begun to follow the recommendation to rely more on student self-reporting, per the AHEAD guidelines but also as a matter of practical necessity throughout the COVID-19 pandemic, as the completeness of students' available medical records has decreased (Banerjee & Lalor, 2021). Axelrod et al. (2021), in particular, notably articulate the position in favor of this emerging practice, and its social justice orientation.

At the same time, significant pushback to this gradual progress has begun to manifest in the scholarly discourse. Banerjee and Lalor (2021), for example, argue that medical documentation is crucial to appropriate accommodations decisions and reduces the perceived risk of 'malingering' by students. This is a fear that unfortunately has been lent credence for some by the Varsity Blues college admissions scandal, where seeking extra time on examinations by students without diagnosed disabilities was reported as one mode of manipulating college admissions processes (Anderson, 2019). Moreover, a September 2022 special issue of *Psychological Injury & Law* was published entirely dedicated to promoting, if anything, *more* stringent requirements for medical documentation of disabilities in accommodations processes. Multiple articles in the issue make this argument explicitly in the name of protecting medical practitioners' role in (and income from) these processes, and Harrison (2022) additionally claims that seeking disability accommodations constitutes a 'victimhood industry' and that recent years have seen 'disability diagnoses become incentivized and encouraged' (p. 227). Other arguments in the issue include the notion that recognizing support needs beyond the most rigid diagnostic criteria for a specific disability is an act of pathologizing 'normal' variance in behavior, rather than a recognition of the ambiguities and continuum of impairment discussed in Chapter 2 (Suhr & Johnson, 2022). Similarly, other authors point to evidence that students tend to report experiences of academic dysfunction at higher rates than the same students actually meet clinical criteria for disabilities, which they interpret to imply that accommodations should be carefully guarded from all but students who meet strict expert-evaluated criteria, rather than that a majority of students would be able to achieve more with more support and flexibility, regardless of the presence or absence of a clinical diagnosis (Weis & Waters, 2022). Across the full issue, a broad consensus is apparent that qualifying for disability accommodations grants students lucrative material benefits in higher education—an assumption rendered specious to say the least by many of the student narratives described in earlier chapters. Their arguments overwhelmingly reinforce the neoliberal and carceral attitudes that students have been shown to face and internalize in higher education, and that present such significant barriers to their equitable access to education: that they are not to be trusted as judges of their own experiences, that their challenges are to be minimalized and trivialized, and that they should always be considered suspect of malicious fraud in order to acquire unfair and undeserved advantages over their peers.

At the institutional level, the gradual increase in adherence to AHEAD's guidelines represents the most significant progress to date toward eliminating burdensome documentation requirements for disabled students, and it is extremely disheartening that even these modest gains have met with such aggressively reactionary responses. At the course level, however, as with time flexibility, individual faculty may choose not to require official documentation in order for students to receive what might be considered accommodations. In one practical example, an instructor chose to eliminate any need for official disability documentation in order to skip one examination without academic penalty, and found that this did not lead to more students than usual missing the exam (Norris & Wood, 2023). While this is a relatively modest modification, and uptake might have been different for offering more substantial assistance in the course, these findings do seem to tentatively contradict the narrative that any student would jump at the chance to falsely claim accommodations if they could. Guidance on UDL also highlights many other pathways by which faculty can make their classes more accessible for all, ideally rendering it a moot point which students qualify for accommodations and which do not; in fact, this is part of the core purpose of UDL (Tobin & Behling, 2018, pp. 44–45). In practice, however, while these individual efforts are better than none, UDL cannot truly achieve this purpose when implemented only by select faculty in select circumstances. At least for now, qualifying for accommodations remains students' main source of leverage against faculty who resist more accessible practices, even if accommodations often do not live up to their full potential either. When even this much security can only be obtained through medical channels that can be arduous and costly, it is impossible to say that institutions are truly providing the accommodating environment to which students are entitled. In terms of the systemic change that is needed in this area, promising practices in many ways still have yet to be observed, and much more work toward broad implementation of UDL and similar practices is needed.

Assistive Technologies

In some of the less fundamental areas for change that students' narratives suggest, however, more significant steps have been taken. As briefly touched upon in Chapter 4, various types of assistive technologies are considered at least potentially beneficial and desirable for students across multiple categories.[1] Dyslexic students, for example, can greatly benefit from computer support and lookup capabilities, to help them with decoding and encoding written information.[2] Some dyslexic students also find audiobooks and class recordings to be beneficial, although they can also be the source of a number of logistical frustrations (Olofsson et al., 2012; Cipolla, 2018). Technological supports like reminder and scheduling features have been found to be helpful for students with TBI (Brown et al., 2017; Leopold et al., 2019) and those who are chronically ill (Ravert et al., 2017). As discussed in Chapter 4, out-of-class access or playback options for class materials are also very important to students across all categories, for managing memory, information processing, and other issues. Students have even indicated that perhaps the most important feature of assistive technology, over any specific functions, is the control that it provides them over how they engage with content (Pino & Mortari, 2014).

---

1   MacCullagh et al., 2016; Couzens et al., 2015; Brown et al., 2017; Accardo et al., 2019b; Clouder et al., 2020.
2   Olofsson et al., 2012; Wilson, 2012; Wennås Brante, 2013; Pirttimaa, 2015; Cipolla, 2018.

There have been a number of examples of assistive technologies offered by institutions as a disability support, although access is by no means universal. What is considered to constitute 'assistive technology' varies widely, as indicated by Jackson's (2023) broad dissertation study of implementations. The same study also found that assistive technology practices tend to depend on available funding and other resources for effectiveness, as well as program organization: centralized, coordinated initiatives from the leadership level of the institution tend to gain the most traction. Beyond simply providing the technology itself, training and support structures are also of critical importance, and current trends see institutions working to further reduce student barriers to technology access, as well as to implement technologies as part of UDL rather than as individual accommodations (Jackson, 2023).

With these trends in mind, a variety of examples can be found of specific cases where assistive technologies have been provided by an institution. There are several studies that describe offering access to assistive technologies free of additional charge through campus computer laboratories, located in libraries or elsewhere (Couzens et al., 2015; Taylor et al., 2016; Sharma, 2022), although in some cases these may only be accessible by providing medical documentation (Couzens et al., 2015). One particularly robust example of this model is the set of read-aloud and similar services provided through the Braille Unit at Visva-Bharati University Library Network in West Bengal (Sharma, 2022); while these services are primarily aimed at students with visual impairments, they can also be beneficial for invisibly disabled and neurodivergent students. Indeed, tests of the use of text-to-speech software with dyslexic students found that it can be used to increase reading speed to equal that of normal visual reading speed for nondisabled learners, with no loss of comprehension (Schneps et al., 2019). This would mean text-to-speech software could serve as a significant intervention for reducing the extra time and effort load of academic work for students in these areas, provided institutions could successfully facilitate access and training for the appropriate student groups. Similarly, as well, speech recognition software has been demonstrated to be beneficial for students who struggle with attention issues and written language encoding, as well as those who have physical difficulties with keyboarding (Nelson & Reynolds, 2015). This could also be a valuable support in which to invest.

While providing assistive technologies to students may carry an additional financial cost for institutions, as opposed to placing the onus on students to secure supports for themselves, in other respects it is also in the institution's best interest. Not only does it avoid the legal risk of noncompliance, providing assistive technologies proactively and from the earliest possible moment of students' transition helps to prevent attrition for those who require them to be successful (Bühler et al., 2020). For technologies to be implemented most effectively, however, may require a certain degree of readiness and self-efficacy on the part of the student users as well; Gould et al. (2022) offer an evaluation scale for these traits, through which staff can investigate what further interventions to develop them may be needed. Bühler et al. (2020) also describe several examples of large programs providing assistive technologies and training at points of transition, including the AccessSTEM program in the U.S. for STEM students, technology use training programs for transitioning students in Canada, funded government organizations and support systems to support technology needs in transitioning to the workplace in Germany, and funded and provided technology for transition entrance examinations in Israel.

Beyond alternative reading and writing methods, other types of relevant assistive technologies have also shown promise. Wearable self-monitoring systems, for example, have been found to help autistic students stay on task with academic engagement (Siko, 2018). Even software that carries no additional cost has been leveraged in some cases as assistive technologies. Examples include using cloud-based document collaboration to remove barriers to writing consultations (Keane & Russell, 2014), or simply providing guidance to free software and permitting the use of mobile devices as an assistive technology (Savvidou & Loizides, 2016). One faculty member even positioned a stuffed toy as an assistive technology, when passing it from student to student was used as a conversation management technique, in order to aid confidence and engagement as well as to serve as a fidget toy (Raye, 2017). While there is no data on specific student success impacts from any of these lower-investment options, in each case they garnered positive affective responses from students. Similarly, another study found that students may devise their own methods of using mobile devices and other personal technology as assistive technologies, especially students who are already likely to have relative technological affinity and facility, such as mathematics majors (Armstrong & Gutica, 2020). Some of the observed techniques in this area included recording class sessions, adjusting the sensory aspects of course material, finding additional learning materials online to supplement course content, self-checking work, making recordings to reduce short-term memory demands and cognitive load, and using organizational tools. The authors, however, also emphasized that in most cases, learning these techniques was a matter of 'happy accidents' for students, rather than intentionally and evenly applied. These types of bootstrapping strategies are also available only to students whose instructors do not prohibit technology in the classroom, and while they may be time-saving in the long run, they add more initial time and effort for students already overloaded with both.

A final, particularly fascinating use case worked to address the meta level of students' other struggles with time and effort, specifically in navigating disability disclosure and accommodations processes: a participatory research project in which students and researchers co-developed an AI virtual assistant intended to simplify and operationalize these intimidating processes for students (Lister et al., 2021). As of trials in 2023, the digital assistant was showing significant promise as an alternative to unmediated form-filling for students navigating disability accommodations processes, and may have significant benefits to offer in the future if development continues (Iniesto et al., 2023).

Proactive Outreach and Intervention

Another need that students have repeatedly identified is for significantly more proactive outreach and intervention by campus units that serve disabled students. When the onus is on students to discover and seek out these services themselves, many students never gain access due to simple lack of awareness or initiative (Brazier, 2013; Rutherford, 2013). Autistic and psychiatrically disabled students have most frequently expressed the desire for disability services, as well as other campus services, to reach out more to students.[3] Information-seeking about

---

3   Pionke, 2017; Anderson et al., 2018; Miller et al., 2020; Anderson et al., 2020; Cage & Howes, 2020; Cox et al., 2021; Grabsch et al., 2021.

available supports also takes time and effort that these students can ill afford, and can paradoxically become a distraction from their academic work (James et al., 2020). Students have also particularly indicated the need for more proactive outreach and integration of disability services in online learning, where it tends to be especially unclear to students what might be available to them (Heindel, 2014; Bunch, 2016).

Rothwell and Shields (2021) describe one example of a disability services office employing proactive outreach, in the form of automatically scheduling students with disabilities into a series of advisory meetings over the fall semester. This model achieved promising results, but only provides proactive outreach to students who have submitted disability documentation, which may miss a majority of invisibly disabled and neurodivergent students who most need this intervention. Unfortunately, other proactive outreach approaches to students with disabilities are otherwise scarce, at least in the current literature. More generally, however, the most notable emerging model of proactive outreach services is in the area of academic advising practice, in the form of the intrusive advising model. While intrusive advising is not necessarily targeted at students with disabilities or neurodivergent students specifically, it is often framed as an intervention for populations at risk of attrition. Bryant (2022), for example, discusses it in the context of support for low-income first-generation students, who 'are typically overlooked as needing additional support as they often lack any visual indicators' of their status (p. 9)—another attribute, alongside risk of attrition, that of course invisibly disabled and neurodivergent students share. In fact, Morris Barr's (2019) dissertation specifically recommends intrusive advising as an intervention for students with ADHD, after finding that severity of ADHD symptoms also appears to correlate to attrition risk.

Evaluating 'intrusive advising' as a practice is challenging, because it is still an emerging area, and as with assistive technologies, definitions and approaches vary significantly by institution. The term is used to refer to a variety of practices across the literature, including: one-on-one advising that includes referrals to other academic support services like tutoring (Reader, 2018); working outside of class with students in a particular course or program, to set goals and develop skills (Thomas, 2020); immediate and interactive contact with advisors during orientation, followed by advisors' regularly initiating contact to check in (Gianoutsos et al., 2021); or advisors monitoring students' progress for indicators of difficulty, maintaining control over students' enrollment processes earlier in the program and gradually releasing control over time, and providing a credit course targeted at building college readiness (Levinstein, 2018). Regardless of the specific form it may take, however, intrusive advising relies on strong advisor-advisee relationships, and its emphasis on proactive rather than passive support has been identified as beneficial for students averse to help-seeking, as well as those impacted by stereotype threat (Bryant, 2022). Positive impacts have also been noted from intrusive advising programs regardless of which practices they entail, from success in a particular course (Thomas, 2020) to improved retention.[4] It is difficult to establish which practices have had the greatest impact, however, given the wide variety in the approaches that have been studied.

Academic advising in general has also been presented as an intervention for neurodivergent students and those with invisible disabilities across a few studies. Incorporating elements of ADHD coaching into academic advising for students with ADHD has been identified as one promising practice (D'Alessio & Banerjee, 2016), and there is the potential for other similarly tailored approaches across different categories. Targeting advising specifically to disabled students' needs is particularly urgent, given that analysis of survey data has indicated students with disabilities generally perceive that they have less supportive interactions with academic advisors than students without disabilities (Zilvinskis et al., 2020). The perceived availability and listening behaviors of academic advisors have also been found to correlate to higher grades for students with learning disabilities and psychiatric disabilities, as have the quality of their interactions with advisors for students with psychiatric disabilities (Zilvinskis et al., 2023). It is clearly possible for academic advising to be one means of positive support for invisibly disabled and neurodivergent students, but to be most successful it may require particular care.

Beyond advising, as well, a few other variations on proactive outreach to students are in evidence in recent studies. These include personalized

---

4   Reader, 2018; Levinstein, 2018; Gianoutsos et al., 2021; Bryant, 2022.

phone outreach to students on a leave of absence, including referrals to campus services and other supports (Naylor et al., 2023), as well as proactively offering meal voucher cards to students who reported food insecurity experiences, demonstrated financial need, or both (Broton, 2023). The latter intervention in particular was found to correlate significantly to increased and more timely graduation rates, and the former study found students who were contacted were significantly more likely to return to study than those who were not. Both cases speak to important elements of any proactive outreach program: the value of human support and connections with the institution, and the importance of supporting students' needs beyond only academics. The broad reported effectiveness of proactive interventions regardless of the form they take, furthermore, should serve as an indicator that any similar, relationship-based programs institutions can create for disabled students would be likely to be beneficial, even if they may need to be relatively modest at first.

The value of these types of outreach to students points to a broader area of need, as well: more holistic, long-term, and individuated supportive relationships in general. Individualization is one of students' primary concerns with all accommodations, and particularly so when receiving help from university faculty and staff. It is a recurring theme across many narratives that one size definitely does not fit all in this area, and the more staff can work with students directly to create individually tailored structures of support, the better.[5] In some cases, students indicate that this is best accomplished by means of a long-term relationship with a dedicated support specialist (Hubbard, 2011; Toor et al., 2016). In others, students also express the desire for more communication between staff in relevant offices, and between staff and faculty, to remedy disconnects they observed between their accommodations, other services they received, and the classroom.[6]

Other types of support appear to be of most value to students when based around strong relationships, as well. While tutoring seems like

---

5   Heiney, 2011; Hubbard, 2011; Pino & Mortari, 2014; Van Hees et al., 2015; Stampoltzis, 2015; Brandt & McIntyre, 2016; Cai & Richdale, 2016; MacCullagh et al., 2016; Toor et al., 2016; Accardo et al., 2019a; Gurbuz et al., 2019; Scheef, 2019; Clouder et al., 2020.

6   Demery et al., 2012; Hong, 2015; Markoulakis & Kirsh, 2013; Conley et al., 2019.

a potential need for students with dyslexia and ADHD, in practice these students report ambivalent experiences of tutoring, with some finding it more effective and desirable, and others less (Gallo et al., 2014; Serry et al., 2018). Some students particularly note that their best outcomes with interpersonal academic support came from personal, individuated relationships and accountability partnering (Heiney, 2011; Kirwan & Leather, 2011). In dealing with their frequent challenges in student housing, autistic students also report finding it helpful to have relationship-based support and communication facilitation from resident assistants (Grabsch et al., 2021). In general, a relationship with any kind of familiar and trusted person can be a critical support for autistic students, and help to facilitate the student's success in other social interactions (Sayman, 2015). This is particularly important in the case of nonverbal autistic students, and those who use facilitated communication (Ashby & Causton-Theoharis, 2012).

Mentoring and Coaching

Another human support, mentoring, is particularly common for students to identify as valued or desired. This has been noted in an especially large number of studies of autistic students,[7] but also those of other categories,[8] including in online learning (Owens, 2020). Autistic students have been found to prefer specifically academic mentoring to any other type, however, and where it has been offered as an option, some reject social mentoring as potentially condescending and humiliating (Knott & Taylor, 2014). The value of mentoring is also not consistent across autistic student experiences, as some express ambivalence about the service (Anderson et al., 2018). Certain factors seem likely to make mentoring more successful for autistic students, such as focusing the goals of the mentoring on practical aspects of the transition to college (Clouder et al., 2020), and establishing clarity of purpose as well as interpersonal rapport in the mentor-mentee relationship (Simmeborn Fleischer, 2012). In some cases, mentorships by faculty also seem to be

---

7   Cullen, 2013; Knott & Taylor, 2014; Van Hees et al., 2015; Anderson et al., 2017; Sarrett, 2017; Vincent et al., 2017; Accardo et al., 2019b; Gurbuz et al., 2019; Scheef, 2019; Clouder et al., 2020; Cox et al., 2021.

8   Erten, 2011; Heiney, 2011; Randolph, 2012; Hong, 2015; Ravert et al., 2017.

more valued by autistic students than mentorships by peers (Accardo et al., 2019a; Accardo et al., 2019b), and faculty mentorships are especially valued by students across other categories as well (Timmerman & Mulvihill, 2015). This can be problematic, however, when so many faculty are contingent and may not be able to remain available for long-term relationships with students, and also when mentoring service is often given relatively little weight in faculty consideration for tenure and promotion.

Compared to some of the other areas of practice discussed in this chapter, mentoring and coaching services for disabled and neurodivergent students have a relatively robust history, and continue to grow. Formal evaluation and agreed-upon measures of impact are still not especially well-established, which limits the evidence basis for these practices, but there are nonetheless a number of promising examples represented in the literature. Most of these can be organized into a few main types of program:

- **General mentoring programs for students with any type of disability.** Even in these, in the available studies, mentees most commonly are autistic, have ADHD, have what are identified as 'learning disabilities' (whether these are also identified more specifically or not), or have psychiatric disabilities. For the most part, these appear to be peer mentorship programs (Hillier et al., 2019; Lombardi et al., 2020; Krisi & Nagar, 2021), although there is at least one described case where faculty served as mentors (Markle et al., 2017), and one where psychology graduate students served as consultants (Button et al., 2019).

- **Peer mentorship for autistic students.** Programs focused on autistic students as mentees, and sometimes also as mentors, appear to be significantly more represented in the literature than any other.[9]

- **Coaching for ADHD, other categories classified under learning disabilities, or both.** These include both the

---

9   Suciu, 2014; Ames et al., 2016; Roberts & Birmingham, 2017; English, 2018; Thompson et al., 2018; Trevisan et al., 2021; Mapes & Cavell, 2023.

employment of professional coaches, and peer coaching.[10] Coaching is a well-established intervention for ADHD that has been in use since the 1990s, although empirical evaluation has mainly started to appear in studies from the last decade. A 2018 literature review of nineteen studies found evidence of positive impact on reported ADHD symptom experiences, self-esteem, quality of life, and participant satisfaction (Ahmann et al., 2018).

- **STEM-specific programs.** Designed to encourage more students with disabilities to pursue study and careers in STEM, these programs typically include those with all types of disability, and mentors are either student peers or volunteers who work in STEM professions (Gregg et al., 2016 & 2017; Dunn et al., 2021; Kreider et al., 2023).

One other relevant mentoring program, which did not fit into any of these categories, is a near-peer mentoring program for students with mental health concerns and a history of foster care experiences (Blakeslee et al., 2020).

Overall, there appear to be a few common key factors in the success of these programs. One of these is substantial training, support, and clinical supervision for mentors, whether through disability services offices or other campus units like counseling centers.[11] Training in both the characteristics of relevant disabilities and mentorship strategies, as well as supervision and accountability systems, were considered a requirement for mentors across most programs and were also appreciated by mentors, especially student mentors. The importance of relationship-building and trust to successful mentoring was also stressed by participants in several studies (Roberts & Birmingham, 2017; Hillier et al., 2019; Kreider et al., 2023), including setting boundaries and mentor-mentee agreements (Saviet & Ahmann, 2020). Where mentors and mentees struggled to develop a strong relationship, this also became a barrier to positive outcomes (Roberts & Birmingham,

---

10   Richman et al., 2014; Farmer et al., 2015; Michael, 2016; Bomar, 2017; Prevatt et al., 2017; Ahmann et al., 2018; Stark et al., 2023.

11   Roberts & Birmingham, 2017; Thompson et al., 2018; Trevisan et al., 2021; Cardinot & Flynn, 2022.

2017; Thompson et al., 2018; Cardinot & Flynn, 2022). Similarly, mentor-mentee collaboration in setting goals and strategies was found to be the most successful approach.[12] Another critical factor appears to be strong structure and accountability for mentees as well as mentors;[13] when mentees were not actively engaged in a structured way by their mentors, but only encouraged to reach out as needed, very little mentoring ultimately took place, even though participants still expressed appreciation for having the option to seek help (English, 2018).

In general, regardless of the specific program characteristics, across studies mentees report overwhelmingly positive experiences and benefits. In some cases these were only identified as generally positive perceived impacts (Ames et al., 2016; Michael, 2016; Mapes & Cavell, 2023), while in others they tended to fall into several specific areas:

- Increased institutional awareness and knowledge, including how to better navigate processes and access supports;[14]

- Improved communication and social skills, mainly reported in programs for autistic students;[15]

- Increased self-determination and self-advocacy;[16]

- Improved planning, organizational, and study skills, mainly reported in programs for students with ADHD and learning disabilities;[17]

- Improved executive function, mainly reported in programs for students with ADHD and learning disabilities (Richman et al., 2014; Stark et al., 2023); and

- Increased metacognitive skills (Thompson et al., 2018; Stark et al., 2023)

---

12 Prevatt et al., 2017; Thompson et al., 2018; Kreider et al., 2023; Stark et al., 2023.
13 Prevatt et al., 2017; Saviet & Ahmann, 2020; Cardinot & Flynn, 2022; Kreider et al., 2023.
14 Suciu, 2014; Hillier et al., 2019; Trevisan et al., 2021; Cardinot & Flynn, 2022.
15 Suciu, 2014; Thompson et al., 2018; Trevisan et al., 2021; Cardinot & Flynn, 2022.
16 Richman et al., 2014; Farmer et al., 2015; Gregg et al., 2016 & 2017; Bomar, 2017; Thompson et al., 2018; Blakeslee et al., 2020; Trevisan et al., 2021; Stark et al., 2023.
17 Gregg et al., 2016; Prevatt et al., 2017; Bomar, 2017; Hillier et al., 2019; Trevisan et al., 2021; Cardinot & Flynn, 2022; Stark et al., 2023.

Given that many of these skills have been identified as critical needs for success through the preceding literature on student experiences, these reported results deserve careful attention. It is also worthwhile to note, however, that multiple studies have also examined mentees' GPA and other tangible academic performance measures for evidence of impact from mentoring programs, and consistently no significant change has been observed (Hillier et al., 2019; Blakeslee et al., 2020; Lombardi et al., 2020). There are many potential explanations for this discrepancy between quantitative data and students' self-reported outcomes, which may have more or less promising implications. Regardless of the reason, however, purely on the basis of students' positive responses to mentoring programs and other students' expressed desire for them in their narratives, these approaches do still very much seem to have significant potential value, even if further investigation may be warranted.

Mentorship programs also have other frequently reported benefits, furthermore, for the mentors. Overwhelmingly, regardless of the program structure or their roles otherwise, mentors report highly positive experiences with participating. A number of specific benefits are also commonly reported: increased knowledge and awareness about relevant disabilities (Suciu, 2014; Thompson et al., 2018; Trevisan et al., 2021); personal growth in self-esteem, self-efficacy, professional preparation and commitment; and similar areas (Krisi & Nagar, 2021; Trevisan et al., 2021; Cardinot & Flynn, 2022); increased empathy, and improved communication skills (Cardinot & Flynn, 2022). Faculty members who served as mentors in Markle et al. (2017) also experienced their training and participation as valuable professional development, significantly increasing their perceived preparation to work with disabled students in the classroom. In some cases, peer mentors were also other disabled or neurodivergent students (Hillier et al., 2019; Dunn et al., 2021), meaning that the programs afforded these student populations the benefits of both roles. Indeed, the highest satisfaction rates with the program described by Dunn et al. (2021) were in cases where students had the opportunity to be both mentee and mentor at different stages and with different peer groups. To maximize the benefits of mentoring for disabled students, the potential of these bilateral impacts should not be overlooked.

It should also be noted that a likely contributor to these programs' popularity is that many institutions have been able to implement them with relatively minimal resources. By far the most recurring model in the literature for mentoring programs is with volunteer mentors, most commonly undergraduate peer mentors, trained and supervised by campus disability services offices.[18] Similarly, faculty members in Markle et al. (2017) served on a volunteer basis, as a form of service. The next most common model is the employment of doctoral students in relevant disciplines as clinicians (whether paid or unpaid is generally unclear), with supervision and support from campus professionals and offices, such as counseling services.[19] Both of these models do cost staff time from frequently understaffed and overworked campus units, which is certainly not an inconsiderable resource demand, but for the most part they rely on volunteer labor and do not carry the additional budget requirements of interventions like assistive technologies, for example. Even in cases with larger budgets, programs appear to be resourced and administered through existing national programs (Michael, 2016; Dunn et al., 2021), or funded by grants and donors (Ames et al., 2016; Kreider et al., 2023). In one example, a fee-based service was provided by a center at the university (Mapes & Cavell, 2023), but for the most part programs have been able to be offered at no additional cost to students, which is generally preferable for reasons of equity. It is encouraging that programs that have been reported as so beneficial have been able to be implemented relatively inexpensively, given that this helps to make them both more approachable to staff and more accessible to students.

Summary and Conclusions

A great deal more work will be needed to make changes to major structural issues in higher education, such as students' challenges around time pressures and documentation for accommodations. There are, however, some potential directions to consider, including evaluating time poverty as an element of need for financial aid, advocating for

---

18   Suciu, 2014; Gregg et al., 2016/2017; Roberts & Birmingham, 2017; English, 2018; Hillier et al., 2019; Lombardi et al., 2020; Trevisan et al., 2021; Krisi & Nagar, 2021; Cardinot & Flynn, 2022.

19   Prevatt et al., 2017; Thompson et al., 2018; Button et al., 2019; Stark et al., 2023.

continued and increased adherence to the 2012 AHEAD guidelines on granting accommodations, and pushing forward campus cultures of UDL. Furthermore, in some less fundamental areas of practice, promising examples already exist that indicate worthwhile directions to pursue. Models of intrusive academic advising already in use could act as templates for, or be married with, proactive outreach by campus disability services offices. There is significant potential in making existing assistive technologies available to students, and more still may be found in co-developing further technological solutions with the students who need them most. Mentoring and coaching programs are already well-established for various student groups across multiple institutions, and they have a record of highly positive outcomes, including greater student confidence in many of the exact areas that have been identified by their narratives as most crucial to success. Though no one intervention will be a single solution to every problem invisibly disabled and neurodivergent students face, each one that is successfully implemented will incrementally improve these students' experiences. This is a worthwhile pursuit in itself, even as we work toward more systemic changes that will address the larger issues.

The interventions discussed in this chapter are primarily aimed at addressing students' academic needs, which is of course an extremely important part of the higher education experience. It is not the only part, however, and in many ways students' lives outside of the curriculum are just as critical to improve, and sometimes even more so. The next chapter will examine strategies for intervention outside of factors that bear on the curriculum directly, and explore what the most promising directions for these areas may be.

8. Co-Curricular Strategies

Just as students' experiences and recommendations have suggested possible areas for improvement of their academic lives, the same is true of their lives on campus outside of class. As discussed in previous chapters, the campus environment encompasses many important aspects of students' lives beyond just the curriculum, especially for residential students. Not only are a student's social life, material circumstances, health, and self-determination skills also important, but they can have direct impacts on academic success, as has been demonstrated in previous chapters. Fortunately, a number of examples of promising practice are available that address these areas as well.

The strategies for improving students' co-curricular lives that will be discussed in this chapter can be organized into these categories:

1. Financial and career support resources for disabled students;

2. Improving institutional social climate and the attitudes of peers, faculty, and staff;

3. Strategies for making social support networks more available for all students, including those who struggle to form those networks organically;

4. Campus mental and physical health care services; and

5. Strategies to develop critical skills and information awareness for students.

As in the previous chapter, some of these areas of practice have been more fully developed than others. In each case, however, there are promising starting points for meeting the needs of the students in these categories, and addressing some of the common problems that they describe.

    https://doi.org/10.11647/OBP.0420.08

Financial and Career Support

Financial Support

As has been alluded to in previous chapters, when students are forced to make their own individual arrangements to navigate a disabling environment, that demand carries substantial, additional, and hidden material costs—which are not factored into financial aid calculations (Eichelberger et al., 2017). Extra financial costs associated with supports for academic study can be a significant added barrier and source of stress for students in college.[1] In particular, in Canada, students with non-apparent disabilities have been found to receive less federal funding on average than students with other types of disability, and chronically ill students have been found to carry the most debt from higher education (Chambers et al., 2013). Students with financial aid packages can find these jeopardized if they are forced to finish higher education at a slower pace than others, or if their academic performance dips, for example due to a sudden flare of symptoms or mental health crisis. Higher education can be prohibitively expensive for many students, particularly in the U.S. and for those from marginalized communities, but there are particular challenges for disabled and neurodivergent students that make material aid for college especially critical. Financial support is extremely valuable when available, as many students have noted.[2]

Beyond financial aid opportunities that are available to all students, there are a few sources of funding for disabled students specifically, although each of these can present their own challenges. In the U.S., financial aid adjustments for disabled students can be available by request, but as with many other services around higher education, students may not be aware of these or willing to seek them out if they are (Perlow et al., 2021). Likewise, the U.S. and Canada also have a number of national by-application grants and scholarships from various independent funders, but, like navigating the accommodations process in college, these put a medicalized burden of proof on students in applying, for no guarantee of any return (Mou & Albagmi, 2020).

---

1   Lambert & Dryer, 2018; Lightfoot et al., 2018; Accardo et al., 2019b; Anderson et al., 2020; Barber & Williams, 2021.
2   Rutherford, 2013; Schindler & Kietz, 2013; Ravert et al., 2017; Jones, 2020.

Tuition benefits for service member and veteran students are also offered in the U.S., although policies and implementation can lead to varying success rates (Hitt et al., 2015). In other nations, there are examples of similar awards as well, with varying levels of remuneration and barriers to entry. The United Kingdom offers disabled student allowances, which can be used to pay for technology and other forms of learning support (Eseadi, 2023), although this aid has been scaled back in recent years by changes like requiring students to make a certain level of contribution before receiving aid (Disabled Students Allowances, 2018). In Brazil, the University for All Program, or ProUni, provides full and partial scholarships to students from underrepresented groups, including disabled students, although it also requires an application process and has significant requirements in terms of income level, academic performance, and verification (de Azevedo Pedrosa et al., 2015).

Individual institutions may also offer financial support for disabled students, although this is by no means universal. Investigating financial aid information online for the U.S. universities with the top ten highest endowments—arguably those best positioned to offer financial support to students who need it most—reveals that three of these appear to offer scholarships for disabled students: the University of Pennsylvania, Texas A&M University, and the University of Michigan. University of Michigan simply identifies the amount of its disability funding as 'at least $1000,' while University of Pennsylvania and Texas A&M each offer a number of scholarships in this area, the former without specified amounts and the latter tending to range between $1000 to $2000 per award. Another member of the top ten, Notre Dame, does not appear to offer direct financial support for disabled students, but does prominently note that it provides assistive technology. Otherwise, information on these scholarships can prove quite difficult even for a dedicated researcher to find, let alone for the average student to stumble across.

Even outside of the most well-positioned institutions, these types of opportunities are not uncommon in the U.S. Careful searching online reveals that they can be found at a number of institutions, many of them larger universities, usually either in unspecified amounts or in the same $1000–2000 award range. More problematic and perhaps more important, however, is that where they can be found seems to be quite unpredictable, and there is no immediately obvious centralized mechanism for discovery of which institutions offer any scholarship options for disabled students and which do not. It is not clear how students would come to be aware of these awards' existence, if they were not specifically seeking out these types of funds at a particular institution. These are also, of course, all funds that are available only on an application basis and usually with substantial demands for demonstrating merit and documenting disability, and compared against the costs of university attendance, the amounts in which they are generally available are quite small for the amount of effort this process would cost time-strapped prospective students. In the case of both institutional scholarships and national ones, the fact that students must voluntarily seek them out raises even further barriers. It seems safe to assume that invisibly disabled and neurodivergent students, whose narratives have shown they are unlikely to identify as disabled or to feel comfortable seeking or accepting even small procedural allowances for their impairments, would be even less likely to seek out and apply for actual financial benefits, even if they are able to. This likelihood is particularly concerning, considering that these are the most common types of disabilities among college students, and they still impact students' necessary expenditures and earning opportunities like other disabilities do. The more students need to seek out outside employment to fund their education, as well, the more their time constraints will increase, and the greater their financial precarity, the greater the strain on their already impacted mental health.

Even so, the fact that some financial supports are available is a beginning, even if much more fundamental change may be needed to truly address the affordability of college for disabled students. Some authors have also suggested potential directions for improving the rates at which students actually connect to these funds in the meantime. Under the current circumstances, of primary importance is ensuring disability-specific financial aid information reaches disabled students, and every effort that can be made to make that information more accessible will be helpful. This work can begin with institutional web presence: not only ensuring that financial aid websites are fully accessible (Taylor, 2020), but also providing clear and easily findable disability-specific information there, to as much as possible eliminate the issues of 'hidden' scholarships described above (Perlow, 2021). Human support for aid awareness and managing application processes is also of critical importance, just as the value of human support in academic advising and mentorship has been demonstrated in Chapter 7. The more guidance students can have in learning about aid, deciding to apply for it, and navigating those often arduous processes, the better.

Career Support

Similar principles apply to career support services for students with disabilities. This is another area in which students have expressed unmet need in their narratives, including for career support services and advice (Gallo et al., 2014), for increased targeted outreach by career services offices (Leopold et al., 2019), and other related services. Campus career support has failed to fully meet the needs of disabled and neurodivergent students for a number of identified reasons: career services staff are often unfamiliar with disabilities (Boeltzig-Brown, 2015), specialized services for these students' needs are often unavailable (Boeltzig-Brown, 2015; Andrewartha & Harvey, 2017), and those services that do exist are often underutilized (Boeltzig-Brown, 2015; Andrewartha & Harvey, 2017), probably in part because of these issues. Career services for students in these categories are not well represented in current literature either, such that there are few promising examples to draw from.

The U.S. National Technical Assistance Center on Transition (NTACT) produced a 2019 best practices document on employment transition, primarily aimed at secondary schools, but with potential for application at the postsecondary level as well. The areas of practice identified as promising for further expansion are as follows:

- Career exploration services, including training on job search skills;

- Work-based learning, e.g. mentorships, internships, shadowing, and volunteering;

- Counseling on opportunities for further education (meaning postsecondary education at the secondary level, and graduate education at the postsecondary), including planning, accommodations, supports, and similar concerns;

- Developing workplace-appropriate skills such as communication, collaboration, and metacognition skills; and

- Building self-advocacy skills. (NTACT, 2019)

All of these offer potential for developing specific services for neurodivergent and disabled students. Additionally, other authors have suggested practices specifically for students whom they identify as having learning disabilities. These include improving accessibility of career services offerings, encouraging student metacognition and self-efficacy skills, including self-assessment of employment-related strengths and challenges, and providing hands-on opportunities to become familiar with working environments—which align very closely to NTACT's recommendations above (Chen, 2021). Other recommendations include creating partnerships between disability services and career services (Verduce, 2019; Kwon et al., 2023), providing training for both staff and students as well as offering proactive specialized services (Verduce, 2019), and fostering disability identity, including by partnering strategically with organizations that provide disability-positive and strengths-focused working environments (Kwon et al., 2023).

At least one practical example has appeared in the literature as well: The Career Connect program for autistic students at Arizona State Polytechnic Campus and Case Western Reserve University (Meeks et al., 2015). This three-way partnership between career services, disability services, and counseling services was created to help connect students to the national Workforce Recruitment Program, which supports employment opportunities for disabled people. Relevant staff in the Career Connect program were trained on characteristics of autism and working with autistic people, including common strengths and weaknesses, and students who participated were provided with support groups, interview preparation, and career counseling. Meeks et al. (2015) report positive responses from participating students, and that 25% of their described cohort were subsequently accepted to internships for career preparation.

Similar programs to the Career Connect program may also be available at more institutions than the literature would suggest. For example, the Autism PATH Program at my home institution, Rowan University, also provides a number of career support services specifically to autistic students, but to my knowledge has not been published on to date. Deeper investigation into practice may reveal more promising examples of forays into this growing area. What is most important for now, however, may be recognizing the unique needs that disabled and neurodivergent students have for career services, and striving to better meet them.

Improving Social Climate

Student narratives offer a number of suggestions for how to improve the social climate of higher education. Among the most common is increased training, education, and awareness-raising around disabilities for faculty and staff.[3] In particular, students note the need for faculty and staff to be more aware of the diversity of needs and presentations that may occur in students with accessibility and support needs, even between multiple students with the same neurodivergence or disability (Erten, 2011). Conley et al. (2019) also specifically notes that when supporting students coping with trauma and resulting psychiatric symptoms, there is a particular need for training and awareness around other marginalized identities these students may be impacted by, as experiences of oppression and discrimination may also be contributors to trauma. Autistic students, in particular, note the need for training for residence life staff on helping to manage their unique needs in living environments (Grabsch et al., 2021). Furthermore, some faculty also indicate that they are aware of gaps in their knowledge in this area and would like additional training (Zeedyk, 2019). Other suggestions regarding institutional employees include increased neurodiversity and diversity of ability among faculty and staff (Conley et al., 2019) and training in UDL principles and practices (Giroux et al., 2016).

Awareness-raising and training are also common recommendations students make for their peers, for that matter. In a number of studies, students either directly suggest that college students should be more broadly introduced to these subjects (Erten, 2011; Sarrett, 2017; Accardo et al., 2019b), or indicate that their peers' lack of knowledge

---

3   Erten, 2011; Hubbard, 2011; Flowers, 2012; Randolph, 2012; Mullins & Preyde, 2013; Rutherford, 2013; Stampoltzis, 2015; Brandt & McIntyre, 2016; White et al., 2016; Pionke, 2017; Sarrett, 2017; Conley et al., 2019; Zeedyk, 2019; Anderson et al., 2020; Miller et al., 2020; Grabsch et al., 2021; Thompson, 2021; Turosak & Siwierka, 2021.

and misapprehensions are sources of difficulty (Gelbar et al., 2015; Thompson, 2021). Regarding faculty, staff, and peers alike, a number of students' narratives also recognize the prevailing ableism of the overall social environment of higher education, and call for consideration and implementation of systemic changes that would improve this atmosphere.[4] Some students with psychiatric disabilities express the desire for a more supportive higher education environment for these conditions in general, which would significantly lessen the severe impact that social stigma has on these students in particular (Turosak & Siwierka, 2021).

In academic libraries and similar campus units, Pionke's (2017) interview study of university library accessibility with faculty, staff, and students with disabilities yields several other valuable insights into how the social climate could be improved. Echoing students' recommendations about other higher education faculty and staff, interviewees in the study identify a need for more training for library staff in awareness of and sensitivity to the needs of disabled library users, especially those with invisible disabilities. Pionke also reaches two conclusions from common themes in interviewees' experiences: the need to empower neurodivergent and disabled users, and the need for empathy on the part of library staff. The issue of empowerment centers around eliminating common barriers of feeling intimidated or uncomfortable with the prospect of asking for support in the library. To this end, Pionke suggests that a combination of observation, collaborative discussion, and user research may serve as a way to identify solutions. The issue of empathy, meanwhile, centers on the need to examine and improve treatment of users with diverse needs within the library, which Pionke notes should occur not only on a personal but also a systemic level: 'Cultivating empathy within the library involves understanding not only our own reactions to the functionally diverse but also understanding how the library as an institution reacts and then taking steps to address both the personal and organizational deficits that are identified' (p. 55). Through staff training, conversations with users, and other methods, strategic work is needed across the academic library to understand what disabled and neurodivergent users need

---

4   Mullins & Preyde, 2013; Gallo et al., 2014; Hughes et al., 2016; Turosak & Siwierka, 2021.

and how library staff can work with them to meet those needs, and to seek out and eliminate the ways that library staff, systems, and policies may frustrate and dehumanize users with these identities. What library workers learn and how they improve their skills in the process may also be shared outward through cross-campus collaborations, and have a positive impact on the culture of the university at large.

When it comes to matters of socializing, rather than social attitudes, there are also issues that institutions can help to address. A common theme across autistic students' narratives is that the opportunities for socializing on campus are not ones they find desirable. Multiple students describe the available social activities as uninteresting and unappealing, for personal as well as sensory reasons, with some negatively characterizing typical college socializing as a 'party scene.'[5] These students do express a desire for opportunities to socialize, but indicate that their preferred opportunities would center around forming social connections with other like-minded students. This does not necessarily mean other autistic or neurodiverse students—although this is sometimes desirable—but simply others who share their interests, are serious about academic and intellectual pursuits, or both.[6] Autistic students frequently express a desire for the institution to facilitate social connections, by offering interest groups, support groups, and other similar student organizations.[7] A few have also expressed desire for specialized versions of these facilitated connections: for example, helping autistic women connect with one another, or helping autistic students connect with neurotypical peers (Cullen, 2013). One way to facilitate social connections that seems to be helpful for autistic students is holding games and activities with explicit rules and structure, which autistic students may find more welcoming to participate in (Knott & Taylor, 2014). Conducting library research is also an area where autistic students tend to be able to excel and assist their peers, encouraging positive social experiences (Anderson, 2018; Everhart & Escobar, 2018). In academic settings as well, autistic students indicate that they have

---

5 Tarallo, 2012; Cullen, 2013; Vincent et al., 2017; Gurbuz et al., 2019.
6 Cullen, 2013; Drake, 2014; Bolourian et al., 2018; Colclough, 2018; Gurbuz et al., 2019; Anderson et al., 2020.
7 Toor et al., 2016; White et al., 2016; Anderson et al., 2017; Colclough, 2018; Accardo et al., 2019b; Grabsch et al., 2021.

more positive experiences when deliberately included socially, even in cases where there are major barriers to social interaction for the student, such as for autistic students who do not communicate verbally (Ashby & Causton-Theoharis, 2012). Curricular tactics can help to improve students' social experiences beyond the classroom, along with other campus resources like formal support groups.

Social Support Networks

A few promising practices have emerged by which institutions can facilitate social support networks for students, especially those who may struggle to find these organically. One interesting approach in this area is autism training for resident assistants (RAs), to help facilitate more welcoming and inclusive residential environments for autistic students (Bolourian et al., 2021). Given the challenges with living environments autistic students report, as discussed in Chapter 5, these types of initiatives could be particularly beneficial.

Support groups, however, are a much more commonly reported way that institutions try to build support networks, particularly for autistic students—although these are not without issues and challenges. Student buy-in for these groups varies significantly, and groups appear to be of less interest if they are designed with a deficit-based focus on building social skills, at too basic a level for the students participating, or not actually meeting the needs students had in mind: for example, providing a male leader for a support group explicitly for autistic women (Barnhill, 2016; Brownlow et al., 2023). Even when these pitfalls are avoided, though, group attendance can be a challenge (Barnhill, 2016; Brownlow et al., 2023). Smaller-sized groups seem to be most valuable, and those with mixed composition in terms of student level, so that they take on a mentoring aspect (Barnhill, 2016). Online support groups may also serve students better than in-person in some cases, especially if they are focused more on basic skills (Brownlow et al., 2023). Online support groups have also proven beneficial for dyslexic students, serving to protect students' privacy and increase the accessibility and adaptability of the group for students' needs (Grünke et al., 2023). Recommendations for developing this type of group include providing facilitators, maintaining closed groups for privacy, keeping group size small, establishing behavioral norms and ground rules, not limiting students' length of participation, and making connections with outside organizations that can provide additional support (Grünke et al., 2023).

Particularly in recent years, however, another option has emerged for institutional support for student network-building: disability cultural centers (DCCs). These are locations on campus for disabled students that parallel cultural centers for other marginalized identity groups, and similarly create opportunities for socializing as well as holding events and programs, among other activities. This is still an emerging practice in higher education for the most part, with few centers established to date, and most of these relatively recently (Chiang, 2020). DCCs may be the most promising practice described in this area, however, not only for developing students' social supports, but also addressing many of the other issues identified in the foregoing narratives. For example, as is frequently noted, the parity of DCCs with other identity spaces helps to normalize the idea of disability as under the umbrella of diversity, equity, and inclusion work on campus, as well as bringing together disabled communities.[8] Other work that DCCs help to facilitate includes advocating disability rights and addressing ableism on campus,[9] including working against internalized and lateral ableism within disabled communities (Kulshan, 2023), organizing advocacy programming (Chiang, 2020; Thomson, 2022; Kulshan, 2023), and facilitating connections between students and accommodations, especially when the DCC works in partnership with more administrative disability services units (Kulshan, 2023). DCCs also have strong potential to meet the need students have identified for disability- and neurodiversity-oriented social spaces on campus, as discussed in Chapter 5. Positive disability identity, which has also been established as associated with student success, has been identified as an impact of DCC implementation (Thomson, 2022), and some students view their role in the creation of a DCC as an opportunity to leave a legacy for other disabled students, making it possible not only for themselves to embrace pride in a disabled identity but to help others do so as well (Stewart, 2023). Other students simply find DCCs to offer a refuge from campus ableism, which is also a valuable defense for their mental health and well-being.[10]

---

8   Chiang, 2020; Thomson, 2022; Saia, 2022; Fuller, 2023; Kulshan, 2023; Stewart, 2023.
9   Chiang, 2020; Thomson, 2022; Saia, 2022; Stewart, 2023.
10   Thomson, 2022; Saia, 2022; Kulshan, 2023; Stewart, 2023.

In most cases, DCCs have been established at the request of student activists, with varying amounts of effort required to secure administrative approval. A number of barriers may present themselves depending on climate, most notably unresponsive administrations, pathologizing and accommodations-focused attitudes toward disability on campus (Stewart, 2023), and a lack of recognition for disability as a culture, or of the need for a safe space (Stewart, 2023; Kulshan, 2023). Successful strategies for overcoming resistance have included campus disability education and awareness-raising, gathering evidence of support and need, demonstrations and protests, finding allies in the community including disabled or allied leaders in faculty and administration, seeking solidarity with other marginalized groups on campus, and reaching out to disability advisory bodies and disability studies programs (Stewart, 2023). The end results tend to vary widely in terms of their structural and physical location on campus, but are able to offer similar benefits to students regardless of format (Kulshan, 2023). Even once a DCC is established, however, its facilities are sometimes downplayed or pushed aside in terms of status on campus, especially compared to other cultural centers, with poor locations and facilities sometimes working against internal care and attention to accessibility (Saia, 2022; Kulshan, 2023). Even established DCCs may find they are often left out of campus considerations for DEI and cultural celebration (Kulshan, 2023). Clearly, DCCs still face a struggle to be afforded true parity with other cultural organizations on campus—but the promise they hold for students, not only for social but many other forms of support, solidarity, and advocacy, is worth the effort. The more institutions themselves can embrace DCCs and remove these barriers, the more successful and beneficial they can become.

Mental and Physical Health Care Access

Mental Health Care

Considering that mental health challenges are common for students across all categories, not only those with specifically psychiatric disabilities, it should come as no surprise that counseling services are often mentioned as a valued and desired support. Students across many studies recognize the value of effective counseling to their success and well-being.[11] Their experiences of using on-campus counseling services, however, tend to be far more mixed, with many students ultimately declining to access counseling through the institution because it proves insufficient to their needs.[12] For students with psychiatric disabilities, for example, limits on contact time in campus counseling can prohibit their developing the therapeutic relationship that they need for effective treatment (Demery et al., 2012; Cohen et al., 2022). Other student-identified barriers to care include mismatches of hours and availability to their needs, the physical location of counseling on campus with regard to both its visibility and accessibility, and the demotivating nature of transition points such as moving from a pre-survey into counseling, being referred out of counseling, and similar (Cohen et al., 2022). Autistic students have been specifically identified as reluctant to use counseling services (Knott & Taylor, 2014), and have found common therapeutic techniques like cognitive-behavioral therapy to be unhelpful (Anderson et al., 2020). Furthermore, students who are preparing for mental health professions may be especially reluctant to use counseling services, as they are at risk of encountering peers from their programs in volunteer positions, thus compromising their confidentiality (Woof, 2021). In general, disabled students have been found to be more likely to self-terminate or be referred out of counseling than nondisabled students (Varkula et al., 2017), and while the study in question did not examine the reasons behind this pattern, the elements of students' narratives above may suggest some possible answers. As it stands, a number of students report finding mental health support that meets their needs either outside the university or not at all (Markoulakis & Kirsh, 2013).

This is not to say, however, that robust on-campus counseling is not at least theoretically desirable, and many student narratives explicitly state that it is.[13] For campus services to meet this need, however, they would require significant increases in funding and support, at the institutional

---

11   Heiney, 2011; Flowers, 2012; Melara, 2012; Mullins & Preyde, 2013; Ennals et al., 2015; Toor et al., 2016; Anderson et al., 2018; Davis, 2019; Hoffman et al., 2019; Cox et al., 2021.

12   Hubbard, 2011; Demery et al., 2012; Markoulakis & Kirsh, 2013; Turosak & Siwierka, 2021; Woof, 2021.

13   Hubbard, 2011; Demery et al., 2012; Stampoltzis, 2015; Toor et al., 2016; Goodman, 2017; Accardo et al., 2019a & 2019b; Miller et al., 2020.

and governmental levels (Goodman, 2017). Nor are disabled students the only ones to identify insufficiencies in the current state of on-campus mental health care for their needs. A 2017 report focused on campus care for students with psychiatric disabilities identified a number of concerns, many of which echo those in student narratives: insufficient hours, lack of after-hours access, service fees, waitlists and treatment delays, session limits, referral process challenges, insufficient numbers of licensed staff, lack of diversity of staff, lack of availability of psychiatric services, and accessibility issues in treatment (National Council on Disability, 2017). Both students and campus clinicians have also identified a need for more satellite programs and services around face-to-face counseling, as well as better integration and promotion (Cohen et al., 2022). Clinicians have identified funding and staffing insufficiencies as critical barriers to their work, as well as lack of awareness and stigma or self-stigma on the part of students (Parker, 2023). A recent RAND research organization report similarly called for considerably more funding and structure for mental health resources for community colleges in particular (Sontag-Padilla et al., 2023), and clinicians in Parker (2023) go a step further and also identify increased financial support for students' basic needs as a critical intervention to improve mental health. Clearly, there may be no substitute for an institutional investment in students' mental health that is at least partly financial.

At the same time, the National Council on Disability report also identifies a large number of promising practices in campus mental health support. These include but are not limited to: stigma reduction and awareness-raising of psychiatric disabilities and counseling services, universal design strategies, collaboration with students and student organizations, suicide prevention and crisis management, telecounseling, substance abuse recovery, and collaborations with community mental health providers (National Council on Disability, 2017). While this list encompasses a very broad variety of practices, many of these can be seen in practice in the recent literature on campus mental health services.

For example, institutions have addressed issues of campus climate and awareness in a number of ways. Clinicians in Parker (2023) also identified stigma reduction around mental health as a critical need in delivery of campus mental health services, both in reducing barriers to care and increasing resources for providing care. They sought to address this need not only by simple strategies like making mental health crisis information prominently available online, but by working to create a more holistic 'culture of care' throughout the university. A promising tactic for doing so, across multiple studies, is enlisting the support of faculty and staff, by providing training and resources to help them provide basic mental health interventions for students (Blokland & Kirkcaldy, 2022; Pierce, 2022; Parker, 2023). Pierce (2022) also mentions the value of faculty including mental health information in course syllabi, and notes that this serves as a form of outreach that may be effective where others are not.

Various promising practices have also been implemented in order to address staffing concerns for campus counseling centers and other mental health services. Some institutions have begun outsourcing for additional access to counselors and help lines (Pierce, 2022), or partnering with local or national organizations for additional staffing and expertise (Blokland & Kirkcaldy, 2022; Pierce, 2022). Coll et al. (2024) also report on community college partnerships with universities, to provide staffing by students in clinical mental health programs at low or no cost. Unique staffing models have also been put in place at other institutions to maximize limited resources, such as virtual workshops on mental health topics led by 'peer helpers' during the COVID-19 pandemic (McConney, 2023). Still other institutions have begun to experiment with deploying embedded therapists, located either exclusively or partially in other locations outside the counseling center, often to serve specific communities or cohorts, increase access to counseling, or both (Schreier et al., 2023). A similar recommendation is to embed culturally matched counselors within campus cultural centers, to better meet the needs of marginalized communities (Quimby & Agonafer, 2023).

Another increasingly common approach to staffing concerns is to employ what Blokland & Kirkcaldy (2022) refer to as a 'stepped-care model': a model in which counseling patients are moved to escalating levels of intensity of service based on their individual need, from screening to low-intensity care to higher-intensity care. Lower-intensity care may be able to be handled by informal interventions, like online services and apps, or by less credentialed and less experienced staff, while higher-contact care requiring more expertise is reserved for patients with the greatest need. This type of triaged, hybridized care has been found to have the potential to eliminate waitlists and reduce counselor burnout (Parker, 2023). The workshops offered by peer helpers in McConney (2023) serve as one example of the possibilities for lower-intensity care practices, and a health and wellness coaching program described in Bleck et al. (2023) serves as another.

Online services and applications are another fast-growing area of development in providing lower-intensity types of services. Positive impacts have been reported for these types of asynchronous interventions for students at elevated suicide risk or with depression or anxiety, and can be deployed while students are waiting to see a counselor (Haeger et al., 2022; King et al., 2022; Rith-Najarian et al., 2024). These types of digital implementations are still at an emerging stage, however, and while both students and campus clinicians have expressed interest in mental health apps, as of yet these have generally not been used or promoted except as a way of triaging face-to-face care—which means they still do not reach students who would not be willing to enter counseling in the first place (Cohen et al., 2022). One innovative example of work to remove this barrier, however, involved creating a service-learning project for clinical psychology students to evaluate widely available mental health apps, and then using their recommendations as the foundation of a major promotional push to the rest of campus about the apps (Stanger & Lucas, 2024). This project was promising not only in terms of increasing awareness and use of low-impact mental health interventions, but in its incorporation of campus mental health support into the curriculum and pedagogy, providing a sense of student ownership and peer support.

New approaches to service delivery also promise to expand access to campus mental health care for students, especially those developed within the past few years. One of these is integrations between campus mental health care providers and medical care providers. Often coinciding with the new construction of single integrated physical facilities, these collaborations have been found to be able to provide holistic care to students, with overwhelmingly positive responses, including significant increases in numbers of appointments, and anecdotal testimony from students that the integrated center itself played a vital role in preventing their attrition from college (Reynolds, 2022). These impressive results are particularly important given evidence that this type of single point of holistic care is particularly desirable and necessary for first-generation students from marginalized communities (Coronado, 2022). There are challenges associated with integration, including merging often different work cultures and teams, but more significantly the protection of students' privacy when sharing medical records between providers (Davenport, 2017; Reynolds, 2022). Still, integrated services appear to hold the promise of substantial value for students in a variety of different ways. For example, one institution found success with providing a 'BodyMind Approach' support group program as a referral for students with medically unexplained symptoms, which proved a more accepted way to introduce students into mental health care who would otherwise have been resistant (Payne, 2022). Blokland & Kirkcaldy (2022) also note the need for integration in cases where students' challenges with access to pharmaceutical and other medical care come up in the course of counseling. If the challenges around privacy and otherwise can be addressed, this may prove to be an extremely worthwhile area of practice for more institutions to pursue.

Another relatively new mental health service approach that has boomed as a result of the COVID-19 pandemic is telecounseling. This dramatic increase has included higher education mental health services, and is evident internationally as well, for example in South Africa (Blokland & Kirkcaldy, 2022). University mental health professionals have identified telecounseling as a critical innovation to address changing and increasing student needs (Parker, 2023), and students have found it a satisfactory alternative to face-to-face counseling and expressed willingness to use it, especially if cost factors are eliminated (Gonzalez et al., 2023; Ahuvia et al., 2024). This is a notable reversal from pre-pandemic study results that indicated much more hesitancy around telecounseling as a theoretical practice (Gatdula et al., 2024). Clinicians have also found telecounseling to largely be a satisfactory alternative to face-to-face counseling, noting its convenience for students and higher levels of observed treatment adherence, although there are some technological drawbacks as well (Hersch et al., 2024).

A few other relevant examples of new mental health service approaches have also been noted. One of these is programs available specifically for students with serious mental illnesses, which has become an area of greater need due to the increased access these students have begun to gain to higher education; some institutions have begun to work toward developing programs with more intensive therapeutic strategies and schedules to make higher education more fully accessible for students with the greatest needs for psychological and psychiatric care (Mason, 2023). Another initiative brought together campus clinicians and students to discuss barriers and needs for care, and from there to co-design workshops for the campus community; this was highly successful, and in the long term resulted in the recommendation to form a student advisory board for counseling services (Cohen et al., 2022). Working collaboratively with students toward changes in mental health care may be a valuable first step for any institution, regardless of what other strategies may subsequently be employed.

Medical Care

Physical medical care is also a significant need for students in multiple categories, as well as mental health care. One particularly needed service in this area is pharmaceutical services and medication management. Many student narratives confirm that appropriate medications can be highly beneficial for many different types of impairments, but also that identifying an effective medication and then maintaining a regular dosage can be arduous processes.[14] For example, side effects of an otherwise beneficial medication can put additional strain on students' physical health.[15] Taking medication, particularly medications for psychiatric impairments and ADHD, is also frequently stigmatized in itself, compounding other stigma that students experience.[16] Stigma and social pressures against medications may be particularly acute for students from Asian American and immigrant families, to the point that they may be prevented from accessing medications until the age of majority (Young, 2012). There is also significant negative social pressure for students preparing for mental health professions, due to professional biases against certain medications in their programs and

---

14   Hubbard, 2011; Melara, 2012; Randolph, 2012; Lefler et al., 2016; Anderson et al., 2017; Bolourian et al., 2018; Giroux et al., 2020.
15   Zafran et al., 2011; Melara, 2012; Markoulakis & Kirsh, 2013; Hong, 2015; Lefler et al., 2016; Bolourian et al., 2018.
16   Randolph, 2012; Young, 2012; Lefler et al., 2016; Bolourian et al., 2018; Woof, 2021.

among their peers (Woof, 2021). For students taking medication for ADHD, there is also the complicating factor that these medications are seen as desirable for off-label use by young adults in college, and students whose peers learn they take them may face resentment for a perceived unfair academic advantage (Young, 2012), or social pressure to illicitly provide medication to friends and classmates (Lefler et al., 2016). Readily available access to medication management services, with a high level of emphasis on discretion and privacy, would be beneficial to many students in handling another stressful drain on their time and energy.

One emerging practice that could benefit these students and others is the provision of on-campus pharmacies. These have begun to be available at some institutions in the U.S., mostly at larger institutions outside of the northeast region (Davis et al., 2020). They tend to be on the smaller side, however, with relatively few staff and short hours, and are often subject to other service limitations like uneven Medicaid and Medicare coverage, limited discount programs and cards, fewer medications available, and lack of common services for convenience and adherence like automatic refills (Davis et al., 2020). As a result of these factors and other design elements, campus pharmacy locations are often subject to financial precarity, and have been found to underutilize opportunities to partner with colleges of pharmacy on campus, or to supply preventive care services to the student population (Davis et al., 2020; Mathew et al., 2021). Greater attention to increasing these types of on-campus facilities, and developing much more robust services available there, could be tremendously beneficial not only to invisibly disabled and neurodivergent students, but to the entire campus population.

More generally, other aspects of medical care are also important for students across categories, but particularly for chronically ill students. Physical symptoms like pain or mobility difficulties, whether they arise from conditions directly or from aspects of treatment like medication side effects, can be significant and disruptive stressors for students.[17] Neither is this only true of chronically ill students. In fact, some autistic former students cite poor physical health as a major factor in their college non-completion (Anderson et al., 2020). More promisingly, however, more

---

17   Bush et al., 2011; Markoulakis & Kirsh, 2013; Hong, 2015; Childers & Hux, 2016.

positive experiences with campus medical care seem to be reported in the literature than with campus mental health care (Hoffman et al., 2019; Turosak & Siwierka, 2021). Students also frequently mention medical care and access to healthcare practitioners as a valuable support, but most of those who mentioned this were actually accessing care outside of campus, rather than through campus health services (Kreider et al., 2015; Ravert et al., 2017; Giroux et al., 2020). There also appears to be less evidence of practical innovations in the current literature in this area than in campus mental health, although this may simply indicate that campus medical facilities are not experiencing the same crisis of need that mental health services are. A few recent innovations are in evidence that may hold promise, as well, such as using de-identified student datasets for proactive prevention strategies for return-to-campus planning during the COVID-19 pandemic (Tanabe et al., 2023), and the increasing availability of campus telemedicine as well as telecounseling, although this has also mostly been limited to larger and more resourced institutions (Hollowell et al., 2024). Both of these approaches have potential value for disabled and other vulnerable members of campus communities, and are worth pursuing.

In any case, as with mental health services, campus medical services must be adequately resourced to provide robust and comprehensive care, in order to properly support this population. If at all possible, as well, it would be extremely valuable for institutions to consider offering on-campus access to sleep medicine as one of these services, given the significant issues with sleep disruption noted across student narratives. Having these types of supports available within the institution could significantly contribute to students' success and well-being, if properly implemented.

Skill-Building and Information Support

While it is of most importance to materially adapt the college environment to meet students' needs, there are some ways that students can also be supported by helping to build their own skills and knowledge. As discussed in previous chapters, there are valuable skills for students to learn for higher education and for life beyond it, which the institution could support by providing explicit training.

Metacognition, developing and using memory aids, time management and organization, maximizing limited executive function, self-advocacy, and stress management are only the most prominent examples. Efforts at the institutional level to reach out to students with instruction and support in these skills could have significant benefits.

Some students also note, however, that obvious self-service supports at the point of need, such as online tools that are easy to find and access, are also extremely important to maintain (Hubbard, 2011). Indeed, while there are many cases where students may need training or staff support with navigating necessary information, there are also equally important needs for information that students can access independently and privately, such as on sensitive topics like stigmatized disabilities, gender identity, and sexuality (Anderson, 2018). Academic libraries, in particular, may be able to help in this area, by improving the ways in which they already support both types of information need. Library staff are uniquely well-positioned to help students find information about disabilities and college skills, and could advertise this service specifically, as well as ensure libraries have a wealth of electronic resources on topics that students may want to explore privately.

In terms of active support programs from institutions and beyond, however, some promising efforts are described in the literature. This is true even excluding practice at the secondary school level, where a large number of university readiness and transition efforts appear to be concentrated. As seen in Chapter 7, mentoring and coaching programs have been reported to have a significant positive impact on many of the skill and information areas that students' narratives have identified as most critical. There are also reports of other training programs and resources more specifically focused on developing self-advocacy and college navigation skills, however, that deserve attention. The programs and resources described include those aimed at students with any disability (although invisibly disabled and neurodivergent students tend to be most represented in the actual populations served),[18] those aimed at autistic students,[19] and to a lesser degree, those aimed at

---

18   White et al., 2014; Nazaire, 2018; Ford et al., 2019; Button et al., 2019; Rothwell & Shields, 2021; Rolander et al., 2021; Holzberg & Ferraro, 2021.

19   Retherford & Schreiber, 2015; Organization for Autism Research, 2018; Nachman, 2020; Bellon-Harn & Manachaiah, 2021; Yeager, 2022; Nachman, 2022; McDonald

students with ADHD and unspecified learning disabilities (Farmer et al., 2015; Russell & Pearl, 2020).

The offerings described are diverse in terms of format, although there are a few areas of overlap. The most common type of delivery method, unsurprisingly in light of the results reported in Chapter 7, is one-on-one consulting or coaching programs, but aimed at these specific skill areas rather than establishing a more general mentoring relationship,[20] and in one case, specifically with disability services staff (Rothwell & Shields, 2021). Two studies also described intensive campus experiences in the form of multi-day residential training, for students at the point of transition from high school to college (Retherford & Schreiber, 2015; Ford et al., 2019). Most other programs and resources were also targeted toward transitioning students, as well, although with less immersive and more varied formats: a virtual bridge program (Rolander et al., 2021), a support program that began in a face-to-face format and then moved online (Brownlow et al., 2023), a free-to-download short book for self-study (Organization for Autism Research, 2018), and a credit course in the first year of college (Nachman, 2020). Other programs and resources were mostly virtual to some degree, including a set of online modules and in-person workshop (White et al., 2014), a video training resource (Russell & Pearl, 2020), and an online learning and support application (Bellon-Harn & Manachaiah, 2021).

The specific content covered by these offerings similarly varies, although it also falls into rough categories. These include:

- **Campus life knowledge.** Aspects of navigating college, including academic studies, living arrangements, social skills including around residential life, wellness, financial management, technology support, safety, majors and careers, and more.[21] Additional related topics include the 'hidden curriculum' of college (Retherford & Schreiber, 2015; Organization for Autism Research, 2018), and careers and transitions to life after college (Organization for Autism

---

et al., 2023; Brownlow et al., 2023.
20 Farmer et al., 2015; Button et al., 2019; Rothwell & Shields, 2021; Holzberg & Ferraro, 2021.
21 Retherford & Schreiber, 2015; Organization for Autism Research, 2018; Ford et al., 2019; Button et al., 2019; Rothwell & Shields, 2021; Bellon-Harn & Manachaiah, 2021; Brownlow et al., 2023.

Research, 2018; Ford et al., 2019; Brownlow et al., 2023). The self-study book investigated also notably covered dating and relationships, including consent and sexual assault, and financial aid navigation (Organization for Autism Research, 2018).

- **Accommodations.** Understanding available accommodations in college, especially in the context of how the system differs from secondary settings.[22] Other subtopics included disability rights in college (White et al., 2014; Organization for Autism Research, 2018; Russell & Pearl, 2020), hands-on skills in accessing accommodations (White et al., 2014; Russell & Pearl; Rothwell & Shields, 2021), and the definition of 'reasonable' accommodations (White et al., 2014).

- **Self-advocacy.** Training in practical skills and techniques for self-advocacy and negotiation.[23] Notably in one case, also the rationale for why self-advocacy is important, and why students should feel justified in employing it (Nachman, 2022).

- **Metacognition.** A number of areas of focus related to metacognition, including self-identifying personal strengths (White et al., 2014; Farmer et al., 2015; Rolander et al., 2021), self-reflection (Retherford & Schreiber, 2015), positive self-acceptance (Organization for Autism Research, 2018), and theory of mind (Retherford & Schreiber, 2015).

- **Organization and self-management.** Relevant topics include self-developing structures and routines (Organization for Autism Research, 2018), executive functioning, and individualized goal-setting (Retherford & Schreiber, 2015). Several programs also included a mentoring component that focused on these types of skills, either with faculty and 'real-world partners' as mentors (Retherford & Schreiber, 2015), or undergraduate student peers (Ford et al., 2019; Brownlow et al., 2023).

---

22 White et al., 2014; Organization for Autism Research, 2018; Rolander et al., 2021; Brownlow et al., 2023.
23 White et al., 2014; Button et al., 2019; Russell & Pearl, 2020; Rolander et al., 2021; Holzberg & Ferraro, 2021; Nachman, 2022; Brownlow et al., 2023.

Reported outcomes from these programs and resources were generally positive, although cautiously so. All types of approaches received generally positive affective responses from students,[24] even when actual student engagement in a program was relatively low (Brownlow et al., 2023). Both intensive residential experiences also saw students and their parents reporting positive impacts on students' life and social skills, including confidence, college and career readiness, and self-advocacy knowledge (Retherford & Schreiber, 2015; Ford et al., 2019). A number of interventions also found increased self-reported confidence in self-advocacy skills (Russell & Pearl, 2020; Holzberg & Ferraro, 2021; Nachman, 2022) and academic skills (Bellon-Harn & Manachaiah, 2021). As with general mentoring programs, however, otherwise results were more mixed, with cases of demonstrated improvement in skills that were lower than anticipated (White et al., 2014), low empirical impacts in spite of strong student engagement and self-evaluation of improvement (Farmer et al., 2015; Button et al., 2019), marked increases in some targeted skills but much less in others (Rothwell & Shields, 2021), and high program completion rates but moderate success rates in employment and education goals (Rolander et al., 2021). A different and notable positive outcome reported in Brownlow et al. (2023), however, was that student participant co-design when revising the program led to a positive transition in format (Brownlow et al., 2023).

More concerning in this area of the literature, however, is that there has been a general tendency toward deficit mindset and a lack of engagement with critical disability theory, as noted by Nachman (2020). This is a complex issue that applies to several of the promising practices that have been described in these two chapters. On the one hand, the core purpose of higher education is of course for all students to build their skills and knowledge, and it does not necessarily reflect a problematic deficit mindset to develop programs to accomplish this goal with students who have a particular need. On the other hand, if it is seen as a complete solution to implement programs to improve disabled and neurodivergent students' skills at overcoming the barriers that higher education imposes on them, without engaging with the need to remove those barriers as well, then these approaches are in fact

---

24   Retherford & Schreiber, 2015; Farmer et al., 2015; Russell & Pearl, 2020; Rolander et al., 2021; Bellon-Harn & Manachaiah, 2021; Nachman, 2022; Brownlow et al., 2023.

incomplete, and situated in the medical model that views students' needs as their own deficits to be remedied. This conclusion is only reinforced by Woolf and de Bie's (2023) striking interview study, led by disabled students, that troubles the entire area of focus on self-advocacy skills. The students' critique of this concept points out not only that this model locates the responsibility for systemic barriers with students rather than with the system, but also that there are hidden assumptions of the 'right way' to self-advocate. Students are expected to acquire the 'stamp of approval' of formal accommodations, demonstrate physical or visual signs of having a disability, behave as much as though they were nondisabled as possible, and make the people to whom they are advocating as comfortable as possible: whether by embodying white gender-conforming norms of respectability in personal appearance, self-blaming instead of correctly identifying courses and requirements as inaccessible, not displaying emotion, managing others' emotions, and disclosing as much (sometimes private) information about their health and needs as possible (Woolf & de Bie, 2023). Students in this study also identified more promising practices for themselves, in terms of resisting these expectations. These included prioritizing their own time and energy, minimizing the amount that they disclose about their conditions even if that means they are not as 'accommodated' as they could be, finding disabled community for support and solidarity, and refocusing their conversations on how institutions could improve accessibility and accountability, and change in order to make self-advocacy less necessary. This important work should prompt us as educators to reflect: how should we respond and set our priorities, if students' low rate of seeking formal accommodations is not a problem for us to solve, but instead what students have identified as their own form of best practice? While efforts to develop students' skills are not wasted, how might we direct the greater share of our energy toward those that are more fundamental, more transformational, and more challenging?

Summary and Conclusions

As in Chapter 7, the practice examples described here include many aspects that are promising for meeting students' most expressed needs, and also many areas where further work is needed to reach the full potential of these efforts. Local and national funding sources are available across much of the world for the financial need of disabled students, but more work is needed in facilitating students' connections to these funds, and ensuring that invisibly disabled and neurodivergent students have equitable access to them. Questions also remain about how much gatekeeping of financial supports (such as an application) is even necessary, and whether broader, lower-threshold access to funding is not the greater imperative than asking students to invest substantial efforts for small, uncertain gains. Career support programs for disabled students may be more common than they appear, but substantial data has yet to become available on how these function, where they are successful, and where they need to improve. Students have made numerous recommendations about how to improve the campus social climate for them, but some of the most promising, like disability cultural centers, face significant pushback and marginalization from campus leadership. The need for more comprehensive campus mental health and medical care has been recognized, and a number of innovative approaches have been implemented to try to address the gaps, but more resources for these services are still urgently needed. While many programs have been implemented to help students learn skills around navigating college systems, the barriers these systems present in the first place have received less attention, placing the onus on students to work around them rather than on institutions to become more inclusive and equitable.

This is not to undermine the value of the existing work toward improving disabled and neurodivergent students' experiences, because it is valuable. As also mentioned in Chapter 7, every positive change and effort to reach out to these students helps, and is demonstrably appreciated. There are simply directions along which it would be most beneficial for the work to continue, and they are generally not the easiest ones. For example, ultimately, interventions like mentoring and skill training unquestionably have positive impacts; they are empirically beneficial to varying degrees, and students appreciate and make use of them, and see benefit from them. It is also important, however, to exercise great care in framing the purpose of these interventions, and how they fit into the larger ecosystem of making change. Helping students learn to navigate college is very helpful in orientation to a new environment, but it does not mean that university processes should not be reviewed to make them as user-friendly as possible. Metacognitive and negotiation skills are valuable for students to learn to support them throughout their whole lives, but equipping students with these does not absolve institutions of also addressing the barriers and ableism that students could use these skills to fight. The entry of disabled students into higher education is not the problem; the problem is the multiple ways in which the higher education environment is set up to privilege only students with certain bodies and minds. Changing these is most imperative, and also most complex and difficult. It requires buy-in, imagination, and effort from all levels of the institution, including those with the most power in decision-making, which individual faculty and staff can seldom directly control. We can, however, work toward change at these levels by forming coalitions with students themselves—such as in the example of campus faculty and staff lending their voices to student advocacy for disability cultural centers. But this can only occur if faculty and staff recognize the importance of the work, understand that the institution rather than the students is in need of change, and are willing to view students as our priorities and partners, facing true inequities and with legitimate concerns, rather than as bad faith actors seeking to shirk work and obtain undeserved benefits.

Conclusions

Sometimes one experience changes a person in such a way that it opens the door to more. This can occur in a negative direction, such as when a staff member's negative reaction to a disability disclosure leads a student not to seek help again in the future, or in a positive direction, as when watching a parent fight for their rights bolsters a student's understanding of their own worth and power. Sometimes the direction is neither uncomplicatedly positive nor negative. Since sitting on the couch beside my friend and understanding that she really could not do what was asked of her, since sitting with myself and realizing that my neurochemistry had failed me and not my strength of character, I have been humbled to find more and more other students willing to make me privy to their struggles. Somewhat ironically, given the topic of this book, this has become more common still since my chronic illness progressed to the point that I began to use a wheelchair when navigating campus. Even we, the invisible, are conditioned to look for the same visible markers of authenticity that others do.

The voices in the studies included in this book echo the voices I have heard personally. Students vent feelings to me that have clearly been pent up for years, if not decades. They complain of inaccessible library resources, which I gratefully take back to see what can be better, in spite of the complications and challenges that are always involved at levels beyond our control. They tell horror stories of casual cruelty and fundamental exclusion, with resigned familiarity. They cry in my office as they try to understand why an instructor seems to consider them unworthy of even simple adjustments to make it possible for them to fully participate in the vital human work of learning, why they feel seen only as demanding wastes of time and effort. Aloud or unspokenly, as others have to their faces, they wonder if they should even be here at all.

    https://doi.org/10.11647/OBP.0420.09

Worth the Struggle (But Better Without It)

It can be hard not to wonder the same thing, though from the student's perspective rather than an exclusionary one. After all of the many difficulties, problems, and concerns that this book admittedly describes, one might well begin to wonder: is higher education even worth the burdens it entails for neurodivergent and invisibly disabled students? I would argue strongly that the answer is yes, however, and with students' own voices as my greatest source of evidence. As mentioned in the section on motivation in Chapter 4, students across studies speak of the pleasure, pride, and value they find in multiple aspects of higher education.[1] Even as it may reflect internalized ableism for students to reject supports because they want to succeed 'on their own,' at the same time, it conveys a more affecting message: these students do want to succeed academically, and to be able to take pride in that accomplishment by their own standards. Their narratives recount numerous examples of what has been good about higher education for them, as well as bad: transformative, positive experiences with disability services staff (Lightfoot et al., 2018; Zeedyk et al., 2019), faculty (Ward & Webster, 2018; Kutscher & Tuckwiller, 2019), peers (Ness et al., 2014; Turosak & Siwierka, 2021), and their own increased self-knowledge and self-acceptance (Brandt & McIntyre, 2016). There has also been empirical evidence gathered to suggest that, although being disabled does correlate to lower work quality and earnings in employment even for college graduates compared to the nondisabled (Phillips et al., 2022), employment earnings and quality are significantly improved for people with disabilities if they hold a college degree (O'Neill et al., 2015; Phillips et al., 2022).

There is ample evidence that, in spite of all the challenges of higher education, its benefits for neurodivergent and invisibly disabled students are just as great as for their neurotypical and nondisabled counterparts. The primary difference is in the costs: for the students whose narratives are described here, far more effort, trauma, and material resources are the price of the same benefits. All of this only underscores the urgency

---

1   Ashby & Causton-Theoharis, 2012, Cullen, 2013; Drake, 2014; Ness et al., 2014; Ennals et al., 2015; Anderson et al., 2017; Vincent et al., 2017; Lambert & Dryer, 2018; Lightfoot et al., 2018; Ward & Webster, 2018.

of decreasing those costs and barriers for invisibly disabled and neurodivergent students, and increasing the equity of their experiences with those of other students. There is clear value for them in what higher education has to offer, and it is vital for that value to be made more accessible.

Students as Partners in Justice

Perhaps the most critical factor in making this possible, at the same time, will be listening to these students' voices, trusting their experiences and their desire to learn, and respecting their expertise as partners in making positive change. This begins with resistance to the neoliberal and carceral attitudes that position students, particularly those who do not conform to an imagined ideal in their characteristics and needs, as dishonest manipulators and costly liabilities. In Chapter 3 of *Academic Ableism*, 'Imaginary College Students,' Dolmage approaches this problem by dissecting the opposed ideal and anti-ideal characters that educational decision-makers seem so often to imagine as their students: newly multi-literate and transformative digital natives versus resource-draining and possibly malingering laggards with 'new' disability diagnoses, the latter of whom are full of demands that will only hold back the capitalist potential of the former. The authors who argue against removing documentation barriers to students' accommodations certainly seem uncritical of this construction. The problem, however, is that neither the ideal nor the anti-ideal student is real. They are simply one positive and one negative way of framing essentially the same challenge to educators: to develop more sophisticated, innovative, and effective systems and strategies that facilitate the greatest possible success for all students in higher education. In considering the changing characteristics of their students, Dolmage suggests that educators 'might move forward by recognizing that an expanded range of expressive possibilities, instead of creating new ways to be inferior, and instead of hiding inequities under the costume of progress, offer new contact points for engaging with the difficult work of teaching and learning' (p. 114). Why, then, should this challenge only be a negative one when it comes from disabled students? To take this a step further still, given the broad and multifaceted range of human difference, might there not be more gain than loss from drastically loosening higher education's rigid criteria for what constitutes 'deserving' support and flexibility?

If we divest from the 'politics of disposability' as named by Giroux (2014), and truly view our mission as one of meeting the educational needs of *all* students, not only those who offer the greatest profit margin, or need the least and in the most convenient ways, then we will find ourselves required to engage in the tremendous work of changing higher education fundamentally for the better. This cannot be meaningfully achieved, however, without giving priority to the agency and lived experience of disabled and neurodivergent students, and especially those with other intersecting marginalized identities. This is fundamentally Berne's (2015) 'leadership by those most impacted,' as well as the core tenet of DSE to 'privilege the interest, agendas, and voices of people labeled with disability/disabled people' (AERA, 2024). This also, in turn, cannot be achieved by perceiving students as defined by deficits, as lazy and passive, as problems to be solved—or worse yet, as schemers constantly looking to put one over on us for their own benefit. Sometimes students are disengaged, and sometimes they engage in academic dishonesty; there may often be more complex reasons, challenges and inequities behind these actions than we imagine, but they are real occurrences, certainly. There are strategies and processes that can manage these occurrences when they happen, as problematic as many of these may also be in application. If we treat every student by default as a resistor or a suspect, however, we do not only lose the opportunity to know and collaborate with whole people, who can offer powerful insight and partnership in how the work of education could be better. We also create the conditions for that presumption of misbehavior to land doubly on those most vulnerable, students who are most likely to be perceived as threats and even potential criminals because of marginalized identities: Black students, psychiatrically disabled students, LGBTQ+ students, and more. Trusting our students can be vulnerable and a risk, but it is also a moral and a professional imperative. In line with the Freirean principle of dialogue, for those with more power to embrace humility, lay our power down, and see our students as equal partners is crucial to the work not only of education, but of becoming more fully human:

Dialogue, as the encounter of those addressed to the common task of learning and acting, is broken if the parties (or one of them) lack humility. How can I dialogue if I always project ignorance onto others and never perceive my own? . . . At the point of encounter there are neither utter ignoramuses nor perfect sages; there are only people who are attempting, together, to learn more than they now know. (Freire, 1970/2014, p. 90)

Putting in the work to release our assumptions and suspicions, and from there being able to enter into genuine dialogue with our students, is the first and most monumental step. All the other directions for change that have been suggested by these narratives come afterward.

Key Themes for Systemic Change

Inequitable Time and Energy Demands

Unquestionably, this is one of the most recurring themes throughout the narratives of students in every category, and one of the core barriers to academic success and positive experiences. University is substantially harder and more time-consuming for these students than it is for comparable nondisabled and neurotypical peers. Every more minor barrier described feeds into this one, and this disadvantage of time and effort not only makes students unhappier and less likely to make good grades and graduate on time, it puts their mental and physical health at risk. Furthermore, while help may be available to try to lessen this burden, having to seek out that help often actually increases it. Many students also either have reasons not to seek help, do not know help is available, or do not even realize that their experiences are so much more difficult that they might need it. 'Accommodations and supports by request, with proof of need' is simply not a model sufficient to meet these students' challenges. Despite the dedication, hard work, and compassion of disability services staff, every piece of evidence suggests that the overall structure itself works for vanishingly few of those who are most in need of it.

What, then, is the alternative? This is where new possibilities have yet to be imagined, and it will be no simple task. How could higher education institutions, as a complete system, internalize the idea that every student needs and deserves support, services, flexibility, and individuation? Perhaps more importantly, even if they did, would they have the appropriate resources to act accordingly? It is difficult to imagine the answer is yes, no matter how creative and restructured an implemented approach might be. To be sufficiently resourced to truly make higher education accessible, institutions would need substantially more material support from without as well as within, at the level of the state. This would also ease the burden on students to be the institution's primary income stream, which as demonstrated creates inequities for the 'less profitable' students who require more resources to succeed, and adds to their already disproportionate financial burdens. It is not only higher education that must expand its imagination, but broader culture too. If higher education is to serve young adults not only as a checked box for better employment, but as the training in critical independent thought needed to navigate an increasingly morally complex and fraught world, it cannot continue to be treated like an expensive, selective luxury by institutions and legislators. The dissonance in our collective vision in the United States of what higher education is and is for will only continue to widen existing gulfs of income inequality, if it is allowed to persist indefinitely. As Giroux (2014) summarizes,

> The public has apparently given up on the idea of either funding higher education or valuing it as a public good indispensable to the life of any viable democracy. This is all the more reason for academics to be at the forefront of a coalition of activists, public servants, and others in both rejecting the growing corporate management of higher education and developing a new discourse in which the university, and particularly the humanities, can be defended as a vital social and public institution in a democratic society. (p. 20).

This is not, however, to say that all of the problems lie outside the doors of higher education.

The Need for Accountability and Support at All Levels

Why do staff, and especially faculty, emerge so universally as one of students' greatest supports when they are compassionate and accommodating, and one of students' greatest barriers when they are not? More than anything else, this pattern indicates the amount of power that people in these roles hold over students, for good or ill, at least in the context of their education. Because of this power imbalance, seemingly small decisions that faculty and staff make in dealing with students can have a disproportionately large impact on students' experiences, positive or negative. This invests faculty with the responsibility to take particular care with their personal biases and behavior, but this is not a responsibility that all faculty equally recognize. The good news about this, however, is that a few tangible and significant things educators can do to improve students' experiences lie in our hands: simply offering compassion, flexibility, and cooperation.

The bad news is that the vast majority of staff and faculty who are not predisposed to do these things are also undoubtedly not reading this book. We see this play out time and again in professional development programming on accessibility and other issues of diversity, equity, and inclusion: those who least need education on these matters show up, because they are already invested, and those most in need do not, because they are not. Furthermore, and more importantly, few if any accountability structures exist in most institutions to ensure that faculty and staff must consider it a priority regardless. As with the inequities imposed on students by the systems of higher education, this is not a problem that individual choices can entirely address. Neither, for that matter, is it a problem that individual choices entirely caused. I would imagine that most faculty who balk at accommodations, insist on pedagogically unnecessary and inaccessible format elements, and even make callous remarks to students do so not out of malice or even necessarily out of apathy. In the majority of cases, I believe the more likely culprits are lack of knowledge, lack of awareness, and the impact of stress from being severely overworked and under-resourced themselves. As I mentioned in the introduction, most faculty are not in the position to witness the real emotional, psychological, and physical distress that their behavior worsens; most students try strenuously to avoid being emotionally vulnerable enough with faculty to display that distress, and with good reason. Lacking this insight as well as adequate preparation and resources for inclusive instruction, it could be easy for a harried, overburdened instructor in an understaffed department to miss the great personal cost of a student's asking for help at all, and dismiss it as the product of laziness or lack of commitment rather than the real need it represents. Such an instructor is even less likely to spontaneously put in work to improve the accessibility of their courses, for the sake of students who choose not to ask for help at all.

The more significant and systemic problem is that faculty, even more than staff, are not consistently trained, supported, and incentivized to facilitate the success of marginalized students, including that of disabled and neurodivergent students. As I have mentioned, even basic pedagogical skills are not reliably components of the degree programs that credential college and university faculty, let alone inclusive and culturally relevant pedagogies. Erosion of full-time employment and tenure continue to increase the time and effort burdens on faculty of all types, and under these conditions, only the most passionate about working to improve instruction for marginalized students will do so. This is especially true when faculty are also not evaluated on this work consistently or, in many cases, at all. Furthermore, the faculty invested enough to devote extra, unrecognized work to teaching inclusively are most commonly those who are marginalized themselves, increasing time and effort inequalities at their level as well. For these problems to begin to be rectified, it will be necessary for institutions to commit to ensuring that faculty are fully prepared to teach all types of students, to investing the resources to ensure that they have time, funding, and support to do so, and to consistently hold them accountable for this work in tangible ways. Neither should tenure, I will argue, enable a faculty member to refuse to support equity for marginalized students, if instruction is to be truly equitable for all. Tenure is vital to protect academic freedom, but should not grant a freedom to succumb to biases and exacerbate inequities. Faculty and staff deserve access to support, resources, and preparation, but students also deserve ready access to channels of restorative justice should they experience harm. Employees' rights should be respected, and so should students', and balanced with great care where they conflict.

Before all of this will be possible, however, institutions themselves will also need to be held accountable for implementing it, as well as adequately resourced to do so. Even as the issues are not fully resolvable by an individual staff or faculty member, they are also not fully resolvable by an individual institution. Lack of standardization and accountability in how disabled and neurodivergent students are supported has led to broad inconsistency in the implementation of legislative requirements from one institution to the next, which in turn creates inequity from the very moment that students select colleges and universities to which to apply. For the most part, furthermore, those institutions with poorer support systems have them not deliberately, but because—just as with faculty—they lack access to sufficient resources to provide better, and simultaneously are not held sufficiently accountable for doing so. Failure to follow through on the promise of education for all disabled people, and all that it entails, is a problem with roots at the national level, not just the local one. It will take change at the national level to rectify it in any systematic and comprehensive way.

The Need to Create Human Connections

Although power imbalances make the issue starkest with faculty and staff, the critical importance of other people as supports (and barriers) goes far beyond them. The support of family members is a powerful asset to students, from academic work to daily living activities to housing conditions—and it is only available to those whose family are available, supportive, and able to devote sufficient time and resources to it. The support of peers and friends is cited time and again as one of the factors most beneficial to students—and it is only available to those who successfully develop strong friendships and support networks for themselves. The large influence of these connections is cause for concern, considering that some students in these categories are so likely to have significant social challenges and family tensions. The presence of this type of support is much appreciated, but this also means that its absence is keenly felt, and may widen existing gulfs of inequity.

It is important for faculty and staff to recognize the tremendous influence that other people in students' lives have on their success, and not take for granted that students already have access to those connections. While in most cases these may be personal and non-academic supports for students, it would nonetheless be greatly beneficial for the academic institution to take a more active role in facilitating connections for students, to assist those who most need it in finding informal as well as formal support. There is a place for work to be done that connects disabled and neurodivergent students to other disabled and neurodivergent students, as well as connecting them to nondisabled and neurotypical student peers, to staff, to faculty, to counselors, to medical professionals, and more. Even at the formal level, another of the supports for which students most clearly express need is lasting, individual connections to people. They need staff members who get to know them, learn and work with their individual characteristics, and connect and coordinate with others to communicate about them in a holistic way. This is something from which invisibly disabled and neurodivergent students would certainly benefit, but it seems equally certain that a majority of other students would, as well, whether they have a known learning difference or not. At the same time, however, advising and counseling services at many institutions seem to become less comprehensive and personalized as time goes by, not more. What is preventing this type of individual case management for students is not a lack of need, but a lack of resources, mainly human but also well beyond that. A major reimagination of the functioning of higher education would be necessary to be able to consider meeting this need, but it would be extremely worthy of consideration.

Next Steps

In each of these cases, as I have repeated, the work is larger than any one individual person, or any one individual institution. This does not mean, however, that individuals can do nothing to improve matters, particularly in the shorter term. High-level, systemic change may be needed, but systemic change occurs through the collective action of individuals. Furthermore, there are individual actions—such as improving course structure and offering compassion as a faculty member—that do make a difference for individual students, even if they may not substantively address the underlying problems. Even the smallest things are worth doing, if they improve students' lives in some way. The smaller actions we are able to take in the short term also have the potential to lay groundwork for broader future changes, as they are possible to implement. Chapters 7 and 8 point to many of these more modest places to begin, with the caution that they should not be implemented in ways that reinforce existing ableist attitudes, nor confused with the most critical work that is needed.

That most critical work, instead, begins with coalition-building and advocacy. Those who are supportive of neurodivergent and disabled students are too often not explicitly identified on campus, but we do exist, and many of us would like to see conditions improved for our students. Armed with increasing knowledge of what most often helps and hinders students, we can turn our attention to joining forces with students and with one another, and using our voices to support change at multiple levels: within our departments and offices, within the institution, in the state, and nationally. If greater funding, resources, and state support are needed to improve conditions substantively for students, then that argument needs to be made to those who are able to grant those things, as well as demonstration of the current inequities at work. The evidence exists, ready to be used; I hope that if this book serves no other purpose, it serves to present and organize that evidence. I hope it can be put to good use in persuading others of the urgency of this matter.

On that subject, although clearly a great deal of research already exists on these students' experiences, gaps and potential directions for future research have also been revealed by this work. Given the patterns I have noted on the overwhelming whiteness of participants in studies of neurodivergent students, there is a clear need for more research specifically on the experiences and needs of neurodivergent students of color. In particular, Black and Latino/a/e voices have been significantly underrepresented in the research to date on neurodivergent students and other young adults, and it will be critical to expand the literature in this direction in the future. As I also noted, there were also several types of conditions that would have been helpful to add to my list of categories in this study, but I was unable to do so simply because of the lack of existing research available. In particular, the relative absence of specific information on students with dyscalculia, dysgraphia, dyspraxia, and Tourette Syndrome is a significant limitation of the present study, and the body of research on neurodivergent and invisibly disabled students would benefit from specific studies focused on these conditions in the future. Although there was sufficient literature to include traumatic brain injuries as a category, literature in this area is also substantially sparser than for the other categories examined, and therefore the conclusions regarding these students may not be as robust or reliable. Additional research on the experiences of students with TBI is also needed.

More broadly, while it is heartening that discussions of ableism in higher education and academia are gaining traction in recent years (see for example the works of Dolmage, Price, and Brown and Leigh, among others), there is still more work to do in expanding on this topic and foregrounding it in more mainstream scholarship. Topics of disability and ableism, while increasingly prominent, remain relatively niche outside of disability studies in much of the academy. As mentioned, another topic only beginning to gain traction as a subject of serious study, and highly relevant to the discussion here, is that of time poverty, especially as it relates to higher education. Further study of the role of time poverty in the lives of college students and disabled people in particular, as well as those who are both, would likely offer a great deal of additional insight, and produce additional evidence about how deeply change is needed.

Bibliography

Abrams, E. J., & Abes, E. S. (2021). 'It's finding peace in my body': Crip theory to understand authenticity for a queer, disabled college student. *Journal of College Student Development, 62*(3), 261–275, https//doi.org/10.1353/csd.2021.0021.

Abrams, Z. (2022). Student mental health is in crisis. Campuses are rethinking their approach. *Monitor on Psychology,* 60, https://www.apa.org/monitor/2022/10/mental-health-campus-care.

Accardo, A. L., Bean, K., Cook, B., Gillies, A., Edgington, R., Kuder, S. J., & Bomgardner, E. M. (2019a). College access, success and equity for students on the autism spectrum. *Journal of Autism and Developmental Disorders, 49*(12), 4877–4890, https//doi.org/10.1007/s10803-019-04205-8.

Accardo, A. L., Kuder, S. J., & Woodruff, J. (2019b). Accommodations and support services preferred by college students with autism spectrum disorder. *Autism, 23*(3), 574–583, https://doi.org/10.1177/1362361318760490.

Adams, D., Simpson, K., Davies, L., Campbell, C., & Macdonald, L. (2019). Online learning for university students on the autism spectrum: A systematic review and questionnaire study. *Australasian Journal of Educational Technology, 35*(6), 111–131, https://doi.org/10.14742/ajet.5483.

Agarwal, N. (2011). *Beyond accommodations: Perceptions of students with disabilities in a hispanic serving institution* (Publication No. 3490100). [Doctoral dissertation, University of Texas at El Paso]. ProQuest Dissertations & Theses Global, https://scholarworks.utep.edu/dissertations/AAI3490100.

Agobiani, S., & Scott-Roberts, S. (2015). An investigation into the prevalence of the co-existence of dyslexia and self-reported symptomology of Attention Deficit Hyperactivity Disorder in Higher Education students and the effect on self-image and self-esteem. *Widening Participation and Lifelong Learning, 17*(4), 20–48, https//doi.org/10.5456/wpll.17.4.20.

Ahmann, E., Tuttle, L. J., Saviet, M., & Wright, S. D. (2018). A descriptive review of ADHD coaching research: Implications for college students. *Journal of Postsecondary Education and Disability, 31*(1), 17–39.

Ahuvia, I. L., Sung, J. Y., Dobias, M. L., Nelson, B. D., Richmond, L. L., London, B., & Schleider, J. L. (2024). College student interest in teletherapy and self-guided mental health supports during the COVID-19 pandemic. *Journal of American College Health, 72*(3), 940–946, https://doi.org/10.1080/07448481.2 022.2062245.

Ames, M. E., McMorris, C. A., Alli, L. N., & Bebko, J. M. (2016). Overview and evaluation of a mentorship program for university students with ASD. *Focus on Autism and Other Developmental Disabilities, 31*(1), 27–36, https://doi.org/10.1177/1088357615583465.

Anderson, A. (2018). Autism and the academic library: a study of online communication. *College & Research Libraries, 79*(5), 645–658, https://doi.org/10.5860/crl.79.5.645.

Anderson, A. M. (2016). *Wrong planet, right library: College students with autism spectrum disorder and the academic library* (Publication No. 10120566). [Doctoral dissertation, Florida State University]. Available from ProQuest Dissertations & Theses Global, http://purl.flvc.org/fsu/fd/FSU_2016SP_Anderson_fsu_0071E_13037.

Anderson, A. H., Carter, M., & Stephenson, J. (2018). Perspectives of university students with autism spectrum disorder. *Journal of Autism and Developmental Disorders, 48*(3), 651–665, https//doi.org/10.1007/s10803-017-3257-3.

Anderson, A. H., Stephenson, J., & Carter, M. (2017). A systematic literature review of the experiences and supports of students with autism spectrum disorder in post-secondary education. *Research in Autism Spectrum Disorders, 39*, 33–53, https://doi.org/10.1016/j.rasd.2017.04.002.

Anderson, A. H., Stephenson, J., & Carter, M. (2020). Perspectives of former students with ASD from Australia and New Zealand on their university experience. *Journal of Autism and Developmental Disorders, 50*(8), 2886–2901, https://doi.org/10.1007/s10803-020-04386-7.

Anderson, C., & Butt, C. (2017). Young adults on the autism spectrum at college: Successes and stumbling blocks. *Journal of Autism and Developmental Disorders, 47*(10), 3029–3039, https://doi.org/10.1007/s10803-017-3218-x.

Anderson, N. (2019, March 29). Abuse of 'extended time' on SAT and ACT outrages learning disability community. *The Washington Post*, https://www.washingtonpost.com/local/education/abuse-of-extended-time-on-sat-and-act-outrages-learning-disability-community/2019/03/29/d58de3c6-4c1f-11e9-9663-00ac73f49662_story.html.

Andreassen, R., Jensen, M. S., & Bråten, I. (2017). Investigating self-regulated study strategies among postsecondary students with and without dyslexia: A diary method study. *Reading and Writing, 30*(9), 1891–1916, https://doi.org/10.1007/s11145-017-9758-9.

Andrewartha, L., & Harvey, A. (2017). Employability and student equity in higher education: The role of university careers services. *Australian Journal of Career Development, 26*(2), 71–80, https://doi.org/10.1177/1038416217718365.

Armstrong, A., & Gutica, M. (2020). Bootstrapping: The emergent technological practices of postsecondary students with mathematics learning disabilities. *Exceptionality Education International, 30*(1), 1–24, https://doi.org/10.5206/eei.v30i1.10912.

Ashby, C. E., & Causton-Theoharis, J. (2012). 'Moving quietly through the door of opportunity': Perspectives of college students who type to communicate. *Equity and Excellence in Education, 45*(2), 261–282, https://doi.org/10.1080/1 0665684.2012.666939.

Assadi, A. (2021). *Masculinity, mental health, and attitudes towards help seeking* (Publication No. 29166779) [Doctoral dissertation, University of Arkansas at Little Rock]. Available from ProQuest Dissertations & Theses Global.

Axelrod, J., Meyer, A., Alexander, J., Hall, E., & Orr, K. (2021). Non-burdensome process: An argument in support of reframing what constitutes necessary disability documentation. *Learning Disabilities: A Multidisciplinary Journal, 26*(2), 11–21, https://doi.org/10.18666/LDMJ-2021-V26-I2-11112.

Banerjee, M., & Lalor, A. R. (2021). Critical perspectives on disability documentation in higher education: Current trends and observations. *Learning Disabilities: A Multidisciplinary Journal, 26*(2), 1–10, https://doi.org/10.18666/LDMJ-2021-V26-I2-10857.

Banks, J. (2014). Barriers and supports to postsecondary transition: Case studies of African American students with disabilities. *Remedial and Special Education, 35*(1), 28–39, https://doi.org/10.1177/0741932513512209.

Barber, D., & Williams, J. L. (2021). Invisible chronic illness in female college students. *Journal of Postsecondary Education and Disability, 34*(4), 311–330, https://eric.ed.gov/?id=EJ1342743.

Barksdale, C. L., & Molock, S. D. (2009). Perceived norms and mental health help seeking among African American college students. *Journal of Behavioral Health Services & Research, 36*(3), 285–299, https://doi.org/10.1007/s11414-008-9138-y.

Barnard, J. D. (2016). Student-athletes' perceptions of mental illness and attitudes toward help-seeking. *Journal of College Student Psychotherapy, 30*(3), 161–175, https://doi.org/10.1080/87568225.2016.1177421.

Barnett, E. A., & Cho, S. (2023). *Caring campus: faculty leadership in student success*. New York: Community College Research Center, https://ccrc.tc.columbia.edu/media/k2/attachments/caring-campus-faculty-leadership-student-success.pdf.

Barnhill, G. P. (2016). Supporting students with Asperger syndrome on college campuses. *Focus on Autism & Other Developmental Disabilities, 31*(1), 3–15, https://doi.org/10.1177/1088357614523121.

Bejerot, S., Eriksson, J. M., Bonde, S., Carlström, K., Humble, M. B., & Eriksson, E. (2012). The extreme male brain revisited: Gender coherence in adults with autism spectrum disorder. *British Journal of Psychiatry, 201*(2), 116–123, https://doi.org/10.1192/bjp.bp.111.09789.

Bell, A. A. (2017). Intersectionality: A critical qualitative exploration of the experiences of LGBTQ persons with disabilities at the collegiate level (Order No. 10269546) [Doctoral dissertation, Eastern Michigan University]. ProQuest Dissertations & Theses Global, https://commons.emich.edu/theses/731/.

Bellon-Harn, M., & Manachaiah, V. (2021). Functionality, impact, and satisfaction of a web-based and mobile application support program for students with autism spectrum disorder. *Online Learning, 25*(2), 190–207, https://doi.org/10.24059/olj.v25i2.2204.

Berne, P. (2015). *Disability justice—a working draft.* Sins Invalid, https://www.sinsinvalid.org/blog/disability-justice-a-working-draft-by-patty-berne.

Berry, K. M. (2018). *Experiences of students with autism spectrum disorder in Mississippi community colleges* (Publication No. 10808556) [Doctoral dissertation, University of Mississippi]. ProQuest Dissertations & Theses Global, https://egrove.olemiss.edu/etd/487/.

Blakeslee, J., & Uretsky, M. (2020). *Preliminary efficacy of a near-peer coaching intervention for college students with mental health challenges and foster care backgrounds.* Portland, OR: Research and Training Center for Pathways to Positive Futures, Portland State University, https://pdxscholar.library.pdx.edu/cgi/viewcontent.cgi?article=1424&context=socwork_fac.

Bleck, J., DeBate, R., Garcia, J., & Gatto, A. (2023). A pilot evaluation of a university health and wellness coaching program for college students. *Health Education & Behavior, 50*(5), 613–621, https://doi.org/10.1177/10901981221131267.

Blokland, L. E., & Kirkcaldy, H. (2022). Campus mental health revisited. *Journal of Student Affairs in Africa, 10*(2), 195–207, https://doi.org/10.24085/jsaa.v10i2.4368.

Boeltzig-Brown, H. (2017). Disability and career services provision for students with disabilities at institutions of higher education in Japan: An overview of key legislation, policies, and practices. *Journal of Postsecondary Education and Disability, 30*(1), 61–81.

Bolourian, Y., Veytsman, E., Galligan, M. L., & Blacher, J. (2021). Autism goes to college: A workshop for residential life advisors (practice brief). *Journal of Postsecondary Education & Disability, 34*(2), 191–200, https://eric.ed.gov/?id=EJ1319189.

Bolourian, Y., Zeedyk, S. M., & Blacher, J. (2018). Autism and the university experience: Narratives from students with neurodevelopmental disorders. *Journal of Autism and Developmental Disorders, 48*(10), 3330–3343, https://doi.org/10.1007/s10803-018-3599-5.

Bolt, D., & Penketh, C. (2016). *Disability, avoidance, and the academy: Challenging resistance.* Routledge, Taylor & Francis Group, https://doi.org/10.4324/9781315717807.

Bomar, R. A. (2017). *The role of online academic coaching on levels of self-determination of college students with learning disabilities* (Publication No. 10601345) [Doctoral dissertation, Texas Woman's University]. ProQuest Dissertations & Theses Global.

Booth, J., Butler, M. K. J., Richardson, T. V., Washington, A. R., & Henfield, M. S. (2016). School-family-community collaboration for African American males with disabilities. *Journal of African American Males in Education, 7*(1), 87–97, https://jaamejournal.scholasticahq.com/article/18475-school-family-community-collaboration-for-african-american-males-with-disabilities.

Boyle, K. M., Culatta, E., Turner, J. L., & Sutton, T. E. (2022). Microaggressions and mental health at the intersections of race, gender, and sexual orientation in graduate and law school. *Journal of Women and Gender in Higher Education, 15*(2), 157–180, https://doi.org/10.1080/26379112.2022.2068149.

Brandt, L., & McIntyre, L. (2016). Resilience and school retention: Exploring the experiences of post-secondary students with diverse needs. *Education Matters, 4*(2), https://journalhosting.ucalgary.ca/index.php/em/article/view/62935.

Brazier, J. (2013). Having autism as a student at Briarcliffe College. *Research & Teaching in Developmental Education, 29*(2), 40–44.

BrckaLorenz, A., Fassett, K. T., & Hurtado, S. S. (2020). Supporting LGBQ+ students with disabilities: Exploring the experiences of students living on campus. *The Journal of College and University Student Housing, 46*(3), 78–91, https://www.acuho-i.org/knowledge-resources/journal-of-college-university-student-housing/archived-issues.

Broton, K. M., Mohebali, M., & Goldrick-Rab, S. (2023). Meal vouchers matter for academic attainment: A community college field experiment. *Educational Researcher, 52*(3), 155–163, https://doi.org/10.3102/0013189X231153131.

Brown, J., Hux, K., Hey, M., & Murphy, M. (2017). Exploring cognitive support use and preference by college students with TBI: A mixed-methods study. *NeuroRehabilitation, 41*(2), 483–499, https://doi.org/10.3233/NRE-162065.

Brown, N., & Leigh, J. (2020). *Ableism in academia: Theorising experiences of disabilities and chronic illnesses in higher education.* UCL Press, https://doi.org/10.14324/111.9781787354975.

Brownlow, C., Martin, N., Thompson, D., Dowe, A., Abawi, D., Harrison, J., & March, S. (2023). Navigating university: The design and evaluation of a holistic support programme for autistic students in higher education. *Education Sciences, 13*(5), 521, https://doi.org/10.3390/educsci13050521.

Bruner, M. R., Kuryluk, A. D., & Whitton, S. W. (2015). Attention-deficit/ hyperactivity disorder symptom levels and romantic relationship quality in college students. *Journal of American College Health, 63*(2), 98–108, https://doi.org/10.1080/07448481.2014.975717.

Bryan, W. V. (2006). *In search of freedom: How persons with disabilities have been disenfranchised from the mainstream of American society and how the search for freedom continues* (2nd ed.). Charles C Thomas.

Bryan, W. V. (2010). *Sociopolitical aspects of disabilities: The social perspectives and political history of disabilities and rehabilitation in the United States* (2nd ed.). Charles C Thomas.

Bryant, S. (2022). The Upward Bound Programs. *Kentucky Journal of Excellence in College Teaching & Learning, 18,* 9–18.

Bühler, C., Burgstahler, S., Havel, A., & Kaspi-Tsahor, D. (2020). New practices: Promoting the role of ICT in the shared space of transition. In J. Seale (Ed.), *Improving accessible digital practices in higher education: Challenges and new practices for inclusion* (pp. 117–141). Palgrave Pivot Cham., https://doi.org/10.1007/978-3-030-37125-8.

Bunch, S. L. (2016). *Experiences of students with specific learning disorder (including ADHD) in online college degree programs: A phenomenological study* (Publication No. 10109983) [Doctoral dissertation, Liberty University]. ProQuest Dissertations & Theses Global, https://digitalcommons.liberty.edu/doctoral/1190/.

Burch, S. (2001). Reading between the signs: Defending Deaf culture in early twentieth-century America. In P. K. Longmore, & L. Umansky (Eds.), *The new disability history: American perspectives* (pp. 214–235). New York University Press.

Burch, S., & Sutherland, I. (2006). Who's not yet here? American disability history. *Radical History Review, 94,* 127–147, https://read.dukeupress.edu/radical-history-review/article-abstract/2006/94/127/30042/Who-s-Not-Yet-Here-American-Disability-History.

Bureau of Labor Statistics. (2023, February 23). *Persons with a disability: Labor force characteristics—2022* [News release], https://www.bls.gov/news.release/pdf/disabl.pdf.

Busby, D. R., Zheng, K., Eisenberg, D., Albucher, R. C., Favorite, T., Coryell, W., Pistorello, J., & King, C. A. (2021). Black college students at elevated risk for suicide: Barriers to mental health service utilization. *Journal of American College Health, 69*(3), 308–314, https://doi.org/10.1080/07448481.2019.1674316.

Bush, E., Hux, K., Zickefoose, S., Simanek, G., Holmberg, M., & Henderson, A. (2011). Learning and study strategies of students with traumatic brain injury: A mixed method study. *Journal of Postsecondary Education and Disability, 24*(3), 231–250, https://eric.ed.gov/?id=EJ966126.

Button, A. L., Iwachiw, J., & Atlas, J. G. (2019). An academic consultation model for college students with disabilities (practice brief). *Journal of Postsecondary Education and Disability, 32*(2), 189–198.

Cage, E., & Howes, J. (2020). Dropping out and moving on: A qualitative study of autistic people's experiences of university. *Autism, 24*(7), 1664–1675, https://doi.org/10.1177/1362361320918750.

Cai, R. Y., & Richdale, A. L. (2016). Educational experiences and needs of higher education students with autism spectrum disorder. *Journal of Autism and Developmental Disorders, 46*(1), 31–41, https://doi.org/10.1007/s10803-015-2535-1.

Cain, L. K., & Velasco, J. C. (2021). Stranded at the intersection of gender, sexuality, and autism: Gray's story. *Disability and Society, 36*(3), 358–375, https://doi.org/10.1080/09687599.2020.1755233.

Calzada, E., Brown, E., & Doyle, M. (2011). Psychiatric symptoms as a predictor of sexual aggression among male college students. *Journal of Aggression, Maltreatment & Trauma, 20*(7), 726–740, https://doi.org/10.1080/10926771.2011.608184.

Cameron, H. E. (2016). Beyond cognitive deficit: The everyday lived experience of dyslexic students at university. *Disability and Society, 31*(2), 223–239, https://doi.org/10.1080/09687599.2016.1152951.

Cameron, H., & Billington, T. (2017). 'Just deal with it': Neoliberalism in dyslexic students' talk about dyslexia and learning at university. *Studies in Higher Education, 42*(8), 1358–1372, https://doi.org/10.1080/03075079.2015.1092510.

Cameron, H., & Greenland, L. (2021). 'Black or minority ethnic' (BME), female, and dyslexic in white-male dominated disciplines at an elite university in the UK: An exploration of student experiences. *Race Ethnicity and Education, 24*(6), 770–788, https://doi.org/10.1080/13613324.2019.1579180.

Camodeca, A., Hosack, A., & Todd, K. Q. (2019). Investigation of broad autism phenotype traits as measured by the 26-item autism quotient. *Journal of Psychoeducational Assessment, 37*(3), 338–357, https://doi.org/10.1177/0734282918768706.

Canty, L. M. (2022). *Chronicles of the 'model minority': The socialization and help-seeking behaviors of East Asian American undergraduate students at an ivy plus institution* (Publication No. 29064455) [Doctoral dissertation, Northeastern University]. ProQuest Dissertations & Theses Global.

Cardinot, A., & Flynn, P. (2022). Rapid evidence assessment: Mentoring interventions for/by students with disabilities at third-level education. *Education Sciences, 12*(6), 384, https://doi.org/10.3390/educsci12060384.

Carter, C., & Sellman, E. (2013). A view of dyslexia in context: Implications for understanding differences in essay writing experience amongst higher education students identified as dyslexic. *Dyslexia, 19*(3), 149–164, https://doi.org/10.1002/dys.1457.

CAST (2018). *Universal design for learning guidelines version 2.2.* Retrieved from http://udlguidelines.cast.org.

Casement, S., Carpio de los Pinos, C., & Forrester-Jones, R. (2017). Experiences of university life for students with Asperger's Syndrome: a comparative study between Spain and England. *International Journal of Inclusive Education, 21*(1), 73–89, https://doi.org/10.1080/13603116.2016.1184328.

Catalano, A. (2014). Improving distance education for students with special needs: A qualitative study of students' experiences with an online library research course. *Journal of Library & Information Services in Distance Learning, 8*(1), 17–31, https://doi.org/10.1080/1533290x.2014.902416.

Chambers, T., Bolton, M., & Sukhai, M. A. (2013). Financial barriers for students with non-apparent disabilities within Canadian postsecondary education. *Journal of Postsecondary Education and Disability, 26*(1), 53–66.

Charlton, J. I. (1998). *Nothing about us without us: Disability oppression and empowerment* (1st ed.). University of California Press, https://doi.org/10.1525/9780520925441.

Chen, C. P. (2021). Career counselling university students with learning disabilities. *British Journal of Guidance & Counselling, 49*(1), 44–56, https://doi.org/10.1080/03069885.2020.1811205.

Cheng, H. L., Kwan, K. L. K., & Sevig, T. (2013). Racial and ethnic minority college students' stigma associated with seeking psychological help: Examining psychocultural correlates. *Journal of Counseling Psychology, 60*(1), 98–111, https://doi.org/10.1037/a0031169.

Chiang, E. S. (2020). Disability cultural centers: How colleges can move beyond access to inclusion. *Disability & Society, 35*(7), 1183–1188, https://doi.org/10.1080/09687599.2019.1679536.

Childers, C., & Hux, K. (2016). Invisible injuries: The experiences of college students with histories of mild traumatic brain injury. *Journal of Postsecondary Education and Disability, 29*(4), 389–405, https://eric.ed.gov/?id=EJ1133819.

Choi, N. Y., & Miller, M. J. (2014). AAPI college students' willingness to seek counseling: The role of culture, stigma, and attitudes. *Journal of Counseling Psychology, 61*(3), 340–351, https://doi.org/10.1037/cou0000027.

Cipolla, C. (2018). *'Not so backwards': A phenomenological study on the lived experiences of high achieving post-secondary students with dyslexia* (Publication No. 10817443) [Doctoral dissertation, Northwestern Nazarene University]. ProQuest Dissertations & Theses Global, https://nbc.whdl.org/en/browse/resources/11741.

Clouder, L., Karakus, M., Cinotti, A., Ferreyra, M. V., Fierros, G. A., & Rojo, P. (2020). Neurodiversity in higher education: A narrative synthesis. *Higher Education, 80*(4), 757–778, https://doi.org/10.1007/s10734-020-00513-6.

Cohen, K. A., Graham, A. K., & Lattie, E. G. (2022). Aligning students and counseling centers on student mental health needs and treatment resources. *Journal of American College Health, 70*(3), 724–732, https://doi.org/10.1080/07448481.2020.1762611.

Colclough, M. N. (2018). Exploring student diversity: College students who have autism spectrum disorders. *Inquiry: The Journal of the Virginia Community Colleges, 21*(1), 21–33, https://commons.vccs.edu/inquiry/vol21/iss1/5.

Coll, K. M., Ruch, C. B., Ruch, C. P., Dimitch, J. L., & Freeman, B. J. (2024). A partnership model to enhance mental health staffing: Lessons from two community colleges. *Community College Review, 52*(1), 58–67, https://doi.org/10.1177/00915521231201419.

Conley, S., Ferguson, A., & Kumbier, A. (2019). Supporting students with histories of trauma in libraries: A collaboration of accessibility and library services. *Library Trends, 67*(3), 526–549, https://doi.org/10.1353/lib.2019.0001.

Connor, D. J., Ferri, B. A., & Annamma, S. A. (Eds.). (2016). *DisCrit: Disability studies and critical race theory in education.* Teachers College Press.

Conway, K. M., Wladis, C., & Hachey, A. C. (2021). Time poverty and parenthood: Who has time for college? *AERA Open, 7*(1), https://doi.org/10.1177/23328584211011608.

Coronado, R. (2022). *The use of an integrated care model to address mental health stressors in higher education for first generation Hispanic students in distress: A qualitative study* (Publication No. 29164213) [Doctoral dissertation, Our Lady of the Lake University]. ProQuest Dissertations & Theses Global.

Coston, B. E., Gaedecke, T., & Robinson, K. (2022). Disabled trans sex working college students: Results from the 2015 U.S. Trans Survey. *Disability Studies Quarterly, 42*(2), https://doi.org/10.18061/dsq.v42i2.9134.

Coulter, R. W. S., & Rankin, S. R. (2020). College sexual assault and campus climate for sexual- and gender-minority undergraduate students. *Journal of Interpersonal Violence, 35*(5–6), 1351–1366, https://doi.org/10.1177/0886260517696870.

Couzens, D., Poed, S., Kataoka, M., Brandon, A., Hartley, J., & Keen, D. (2015). Support for students with hidden disabilities in universities: A case study. *International Journal of Disability, Development and Education, 62*(1), 24–41, https://doi.org/10.1080/1034912X.2014.984592.

Cox, B. E., Edelstein, J., Brogdon, B., & Roy, A. (2021). Navigating challenges to facilitate success for college students with autism. *Journal of Higher Education, 92*(2), 252–278, https://doi.org/10.1080/00221546.2020.1798203.

Cox, B. E., Thompson, K., Anderson, A., Mintz, A., Locks, T., Morgan, L., Edelstein, J., & Wolz, A. (2017). College experiences for students with autism spectrum disorder: Personal identity, public disclosure, and institutional support. *Journal of College Student Development, 58*(1), 71–87, https://doi.org/10.1353/csd.2017.0004.

Crenshaw, K. (1991). Mapping the margins: Intersectionality, identity politics, and violence against women of color. *Stanford Law Review, 43*(6), 1241–1299, https://doi.org/10.2307/1229039.

Cullen, J. A. (2013). *Perspectives of college students with asperger's syndrome* (Publication No. 3574040) [Doctoral dissertation, Widener University]. ProQuest Dissertations & Theses Global.

Cullen, J. A. (2015). The needs of college students with autism spectrum disorders and Asperger's Syndrome. *Journal of Postsecondary Education and Disability, 28*(1), 89–101.

D'Alessio, K. A., & Banerjee, M. (2016). Academic advising as an intervention for college students with ADHD. *Journal of Postsecondary Education and Disability, 29*(2), 109–121.

Daffner, M. S., DuPaul, G. J., Anastopoulos, A. D., & Weyandt, L. L. (2022). From orientation to graduation: Predictors of academic success for freshmen with ADHD. *Journal of Postsecondary Education & Disability, 35*(2), 113–130, https://eric.ed.gov/?id=EJ1066322.

Daniels, J. R., & Geiger, T. J. (2010). Universal Design and LGBTQ (lesbian, gay, transgender, bisexual, and queer) issues: Creating equal access and opportunities for success. Paper presented at the Annual Meeting of the Association for the Study of Higher Education. Educational Research Information Center, https://eric.ed.gov/?id=ED530463.

Davenport, R. G. (2017). The integration of health and counseling services on college campuses: Is there a risk in maintaining student patients' privacy? *Journal of College Student Psychotherapy, 31*(4), 268–280, https://doi.org/10.1080/87568225.2017.1364147.

Davis, J., Traweek, C., & Irwin, A. N. (2020). Community pharmacies embedded within student health centers on college and university campuses: A cross-sectional survey. *Journal of the American Pharmacists Association, 60*(6), e184–e189, https://doi.org/10.1016/j.japh.2020.06.020.

Davis, L. J. (2015). Enabling acts: The hidden story of how the Americans with Disabilities Act gave the largest us minority its rights. Beacon Press.

Davis, R. V. (2019). *The role of self-empowerment in academic success in higher education after a traumatic brain injury: A case study* (Publication No. 13884844) [Doctoral dissertation, Saint Joseph's University]. ProQuest Dissertations & Theses Global.

de Azevedo Pedrosa, S.M.P., de Figueiredo-da-Costa, A.V., de Lima, C.O., da Fonseca Ribeiro, F.N. (2015). PROUNI in Brazil: Advancement for social and economic justice? In E. Brown (Ed.), *Poverty, class, and schooling: Global perspectives on economic justice and educational equity* (pp. 213–232). Information Age Publishing.

De Vries, A. L. C., Noens, I. L. J., Cohen-Kettenis, P., Van Berckelaer-Onnes, I. A., & Doreleijers, T. A. (2010). Autism spectrum disorders in gender dysphoric children and adolescents. *Journal of Autism and Developmental Disorders, 40*(8), 930–936, https://doi.org/10.1007/s10803-010-0935-9.

Demery, R., Thirlaway, K., & Mercer, J. (2012). The experiences of university students with a mood disorder. *Disability and Society, 27*(4), 519–533, https://doi.org/10.1080/09687599.2012.662827.

Disabled Students Allowances. (2018). *Education Journal,* (340), 33.

Disability Studies in Education SIG (n.d.). 'DSE tenets & approaches.' *American Educational Research Association (AERA).* Retrieved June 13, 2024, from https://www.aera.net/SIG143/Who-We-Are.

Dizon, J. P. M., Enoch-Stevens, T., & Huerta, A. H. (2022). Carcerality and education: Toward a relational theory of risk in educational institutions. *American Behavioral Scientist, 66*(10), 1319–1341, https://doi.org/10.1177/00027642211054828.

Doikou-Avlidou, M. (2015). The educational, social and emotional experiences of students with dyslexia: The perspective of postsecondary education students. *International Journal of Special Education, 30*(1), 132–145, https://internationalsped.com/ijse/issue/view/15.

Dolmage, J. (2018). *Disabled upon arrival: Eugenics, immigration, and the construction of race and disability.* The Ohio State University Press, https://doi.org/10.2307/j.ctv1h45mm5.

Dolmage, J. T. (2017). *Academic ableism: Disability and higher education.* University of Michigan Press, https://doi.org/10.3998/mpub.9708722.

Downing, J. (2014). 'Obstacles to my learning': A mature-aged student with autism describes his experience in a fully online course. *International Studies in Widening Participation, 1*(1), 15–27, http://hdl.handle.net/1959.13/1433961.

Drake, S. (2014). College experience of academically successful students with autism. *Journal of Autism, 1*(5), https://doi.org/10.7243/2054-992x-1-5.

Dunn, C., Shannon, D., McCullough, B., Jenda, O., Qazi, M., & Pettis, C. (2021). A mentoring bridge model for students with disabilities in science, technology, engineering, and mathematics. *Journal of Postsecondary Education and Disability, 34*(2), 163–177.

Dunn, D. S., & Andrews, E. E. (2015). Person-first and identity-first language: Developing psychologists' cultural competence using disability language. *The American Psychologist; Am Psychol, 70*(3), 255–264, https://doi.org/10.1037/a0038636.

Edwards, R. A. R. (2001). 'Speech has an extraordinary humanizing power': Horace Mann and the problem of nineteenth-century American Deaf education. In P. K. Longmore, & L. Umansky (Eds.), *The new disability history: American perspectives* (pp. 58–82). New York University Press.

Eichelberger, B., Mattioli, H., & Foxhoven, R. (2017). Uncovering barriers to financial capability: Underrepresented students' access to financial resources. *Journal of Student Financial Aid, 47*(3), https://doi.org/10.55504/0884-9153.1634.

English, L. (2018). Supporting the transition of autistic students into university life: Reflections on a specialist peer mentoring scheme. *Good Autism Practice, 19*(1), 63–67.

Ennals, P., Fossey, E., & Howie, L. (2015). Postsecondary study and mental ill-health: A meta-synthesis of qualitative research exploring students' lived experiences. *Journal of Mental Health, 24*(2), 111–119, https://doi.org/10.3109/09638237.2015.1019052.

Erten, O. (2011). Facing challenges: Experiences of young women with disabilities attending a Canadian university. *Journal of Postsecondary Education and Disability, 24*(2), 101–114, https://eric.ed.gov/?id=EJ943697.

Eseadi, C. (2023). Enhancing educational and career prospects: A comprehensive analysis of institutional support for students with specific learning disabilities. *International Journal of Research in Counseling and Education, 7*(1), 1–7.

Everhart, N., & Escobar, K. L. (2018). Conceptualizing the information seeking of college students on the autism spectrum through participant viewpoint ethnography. *Library and Information Science Research, 40*(3–4), 269–276, https://doi.org/10.1016/j.lisr.2018.09.009.

Farmer, J. L., Allsopp, D. H., & Ferron, J. M. (2015). Impact of the personal strengths program on self-determination levels of college students with LD and/or ADHD. *Learning Disability Quarterly, 38*(3), 145–159, https://doi.org/10.1177/0731948714526998.

Fedele, D. A., Lefler, E. K., Hartung, C. M., & Canu, W. H. (2012). Sex differences in the manifestation of ADHD in emerging adults. *Journal of Attention Disorders, 16*(2), 109–117, https://doi.org/10.1177/1087054710374596.

Fleischer, A. S. (2012). Alienation and struggle: Everyday student-life of three male students with Asperger Syndrome. *Scandinavian Journal of Disability Research, 14*(2), 177–194, https://doi.org/10.1080/15017419.2011.558236.

Fleischer, A. S., Adolfsson, M., & Granlund, M. (2013). Students with disabilities in higher education—Perceptions of support needs and received support: A pilot study. *International Journal of Rehabilitation Research, 36*(4), 330–338, https://doi.org/10.1097/MRR.0b013e328362491c.

Fleischer, D., & Zames, F. (2011). *The disability rights movement: From charity to confrontation*. Temple University Press.

Fletcher, J. M., Lyon, G. R., Fuchs, L. S., & Barnes, M. A. (2018). Classification and definition of learning disabilities: The problem of identification. In H. L. Swanson, K. R. Harris & S. Graham (Eds.), *Handbook of learning disabilities* (pp. 33–50). Guilford Publications.

Flowers, L. (2012). *Navigating and accessing higher education: The experiences of community college students with attention deficit hyperactivity disorder* (Publication No. 3542247) [Doctoral dissertation, University of Southern California]. ProQuest Dissertations & Theses Global, https://doi.org/10.25549/usctheses-c3-67634.

Ford, J. W., Wenner, J. A., & Murphy, V. (2019). The effects of completing PREP Academy: A university-based transition project for students with disabilities (practice brief). *Journal of Postsecondary Education and Disability, 32*(1), 83–90, https://eric.ed.gov/?id=EJ1217450.

Freire, P. (2014). *Pedagogy of the oppressed* (M.B. Ramos, Trans., thirtieth anniversary edition). Bloomsbury. (Original work published 1970)

Fuller, G. (2023). *A qualitative study of ableism on the postsecondary campus* (Publication No. 30638886) [Doctoral dissertation, University of San Francisco]. ProQuest Dissertations & Theses Global, https://repository.usfca.edu/cgi/viewcontent.cgi?article=1660&context=diss.

Functioning labels harm autistic people. (2021, December 9). Autistic Self Advocacy Network, https://autisticadvocacy.org/2021/12/functioning-labels-harm-autistic-people/.

Gabel, S. (2005). 'Introduction: Disability studies in education.' In S. Gabel (Ed.), *Disability studies in education: Readings in theory and method* (pp. 1–20). Peter Lang.

Gallo, M. P., Mahar, P., & Chalmers, L. (2014). College student's perceptions of living and learning with attention deficit hyperactivity disorder (ADHD). *The Journal of Special Education Apprenticeship, 3*(2), 1–12, https://doi.org/10.58729/2167-3454.1037 https://scholarworks.lib.csusb.edu/josea/vol3/iss2/2.

Gatdula, N., Costa, C. B., Mayra S. Rascón, Deckers, C. M., & Bird, M. (2024). College students' perceptions of telemental health to address their mental health needs. *Journal of American College Health, 72*(2), 515–521, https://doi.org/10.1080/07448481.2022.2047697.

Gelbar, N. W., Shefcyk, A., & Reichow, B. (2015). A comprehensive survey of current and former college students with autism spectrum disorders. *Yale Journal of Biology and Medicine, 88*, 45–68, https://www.ncbi.nlm.nih.gov/pmc/articles/PMC4345538/.

Gelbar, N. W., Smith, I., & Reichow, B. (2014). Systematic review of articles describing experience and supports of individuals with autism enrolled in college and university programs. *Journal of Autism and Developmental Disorders, 44*, 2593–2601, https://doi.org/10.1007/s10803-014-2135-5.

Gianoutsos, D., White, A., Smith, B., & Stella, N. (2021). Path to success: Examining a multifaceted retention model for major pathways students at a large, diverse research university. *Journal of Higher Education Theory & Practice, 21*(2), 111–123, https://doi.org/10.33423/jhetp.v21i2.4123.

Gibbs, E. L., Kass, A. E., Eichen, D. M., Fitzsimmons-Craft, E., Trockel, M., Wilfley, D. E., & Taylor, C. B. (2016). Attention-deficit/hyperactivity disorder–specific stimulant misuse, mood, anxiety, and stress in college-age women at high risk for or with eating disorders. *Journal of American College Health, 64*(4), 300–308, https://doi.org/10.1080/07448481.2016.1138477.

Giroux, C. M., Carter, L., & Corkett, J. (2020). An exploration of quality of life among Ontario postsecondary students living with the chronic illness Ehlers-Danlos syndrome. *The Canadian Journal for the Scholarship of Teaching and Learning, 11*(1), https://doi.org/10.5206/cjsotl-rcacea.2020.1.10766.

Giroux, C. M., Corkett, J. K., & Carter, L. M. (2016). The academic and psychosocial impacts of Ehlers-Danlos syndrome on postsecondary students: An integrative review of the literature. *Journal of Postsecondary Education and Disability, 29*(4), 407–418, https://eric.ed.gov/?id=EJ1133767.

Giroux, H. A. (2011). *On critical pedagogy*. Continuum, https://doi.org/10.5040/9781350145016.

Giroux, H. A. (2014). *Neoliberalism's war on higher education*. Haymarket Books.

Giurge, L. M., Whillans, A. V., & West, C. (2020). Why time poverty matters for individuals, organisations and nations. *Nature Human Behaviour, 4*(10), 993–1003, https://doi.org/10.1038/s41562-020-0920-z.

Gleeson, B. (1999). *Geographies of disability*. Routledge, https://doi.org/10.4324/9780203021217.

Gonzalez, J. E., Ramclam, A., Moelbak, R., & Roche, M. (2023). The transition to telepsychology during the COVID-19 pandemic: College student and counselor acceptability perceptions and attitudes. *Journal of College Student Psychotherapy, 37*(4), 301–317, https://doi.org/10.1080/87568225.2022.2029688.

Goodman, L. (2017). Mental health on university campuses and the needs of students they seek to serve. *Building Healthy Academic Communities Journal, 1*(2), 31–44, https://doi.org/10.18061/bhac.v1i2.6056.

Gottschall, K., & Young, D. C. (2017). Female students with acquired brain injury: The post-secondary experience. *Transformative Dialogues: Teaching & Learning Journal, 9*(3), 1–14, https://journals.psu.edu/td/article/view/1003.

Gould, R., Heider, A., Harris, S. P., Jones, R., Peters, J., Eisenberg, Y., & Caldwell, K. (2022). Self-determination and quality indicators for assistive technology in postsecondary education. *Journal of Postsecondary Education & Disability, 35*(1), 45–80.

Grabsch, D. K., Melton, H., & Gilson, C. B. (2021). Understanding the expectations of students with autism to increase satisfaction with the on-campus living experience. *The Journal of College and University Student Housing, 47*(2), 24–43, https://www.acuho-i.org/knowledge-resources/journal-of-college-university-student-housing/archived-issues.

Graves, L., Asunda, P. A., Plant, S. J., & Goad, C. (2011). Asynchronous online access as an accommodation on students with learning disabilities and/or attention-deficit hyperactivity disorders in postsecondary STEM courses. *Journal of Postsecondary Education and Disability, 24*(4), 317–330, https://eric.ed.gov/?id=EJ966132.

Gray, J. P. (2021). Slow writing: Student perspectives on time and writing in first-year composition courses. *Currents in Teaching & Learning, 13*(1), 39–47.

Gray, S. A., Fettes, P., Woltering, S., Mawjee, K., & Tannock, R. (2016). Symptom manifestation and impairments in college students with ADHD. *Journal of Learning Disabilities, 49*(6), 616–630, https://doi.org/10.1177/0022219415576523.

Gregg, N., Galyardt, A., Wolfe, G., Moon, N., & Todd, R. (2017). Virtual mentoring and persistence in stem for students with disabilities. *Career Development and Transition for Exceptional Individuals, 40*(4), 205–214, https://doi.org/10.1177/2165143416651717.

Gregg, N., Wolfe, G., Jones, S., Todd, R., Moon, N., & Langston, C. (2016). STEM e-mentoring and community college students with disabilities. *Journal of Postsecondary Education & Disability, 29*(1), 47–63, https://eric.ed.gov/?id=EJ1107474.

Grimes, S., Southgate, E., Scevak, J., & Buchanan, R. (2020). University student experiences of disability and the influence of stigma on institutional non-disclosure and learning. *Journal of Postsecondary Education and Disability, 33*(1), 23–37, https://eric.ed.gov/?id=EJ1273678.

Grünke, M., Hammes-Schmitz, E., Nobel, K., Ramacher-Faasen, N., Stallmann, T., Apel, K., Faasen, J., & Faasen, R. (2023). Digital self-help groups for college students with dyslexia: What they can provide to young people with substantial difficulties in reading and spelling on their path through higher education. *Insights into Learning Disabilities, 20*(1), 51–63, https://files.eric.ed.gov/fulltext/EJ1379971.pdf., https://eric.ed.gov/?id=EJ1379971.

Gurbuz, E., Hanley, M., & Riby, D. M. (2019). University students with autism: the social and academic experiences of university in the UK. *Journal of Autism and Developmental Disorders, 49*(2), 617–631, https://doi.org/10.1007/s10803-018-3741-4.

Habib, L., Berget, G., Sandnes, F. E., Sanderson, N., Kahn, P., Fagernes, S., & Olcay, A. (2012). Dyslexic students in higher education and virtual learning environments: An exploratory study. *Journal of Computer Assisted Learning, 28*(6), 574–584, https://doi.org/10.1111/j.1365-2729.2012.00486.x.

Hadley, W. (2017). The four-year college experience of one student with multiple learning disabilities. *College Student Journal, 51*(1), 19–28.

Hadley, W. M., & Satterfield, J. W. (2013). Are university students with learning disabilities getting the help they need? *Journal of the First-Year Experience & Students in Transition, 25*(1), 113–124.

Haeger, J. A., Davis, C. H., & Levin, M. E. (2022). Utilizing ACT daily as a self-guided app for clients waiting for services at a college counseling center: A pilot study. *Journal of American College Health, 70*(3), 742–749, https://doi.org/10.1080/07448481.2020.1763366.

Han, M., & Pong, H. (2015). Mental health help-seeking behaviors among Asian American community college students: The effect of stigma, cultural barriers, and acculturation. *Journal of College Student Development, 56*(1), 1–14, https://doi.org/10.1353/csd.2015.0001.

Harn, M., Azios, J., Azios, M., & Smith, D. (2019). The lived experience of college students with autism spectrum disorder: A phenomenological study. *College Student Journal, 53*(4), 450–464.

Harrell, E. (2017). *Crime against persons with disabilities, 2009–2015—Statistical tables.* Bureau of Justice Statistics, https://bjs.ojp.gov/content/pub/pdf/capd0915st.pdf.

Harrison, A. G. (2022). Attention deficit hyperactivity disorder, learning disorders, and other incentivized diagnoses—A special issue for psychologists. *Psychological Injury and Law, 15*(3), 227–235, https://doi.org/10.1007/s12207-022-09460-2.

Harry, B., & Klingner, J. K. (2006). *Why are so many minority students in special education? Understanding race & disability in schools.* Teachers College Press.

Heindel, A. J. (2015). *A phenomenological study of the experiences of higher education students with disabilities with online coursework* (Publication No. AAI3617345) [Doctoral dissertation, University of South Florida]. APA PsycInfo, https://digitalcommons.usf.edu/etd/5037/.

Heiney, E. P. (2011). *Factors within the post-secondary education environment that positively impact the academic success of college students with ADHD* (Publication No. 3444116) [Doctoral dissertation, Spalding University]. ProQuest Dissertations & Theses Global.

Hersch, E., Cohen, K. A., Saklecha, A., Williams, K. D. A., Tan, Y., & Lattie, E. G. (2024). Remote-delivered services during COVID-19: A mixed-methods survey of college counseling center clinicians. *Journal of American College Health, 72*(2), 423–431, https://doi.org/10.1080/07448481.2022.2038178.

Hewett, R., Douglas, G., McLinden, M., & Keil, S. (2017). Developing an inclusive learning environment for students with visual impairment in higher education: Progressive mutual accommodation and learner experiences in the United Kingdom. *European Journal of Special Needs Education, 32*(1), 89–109, https://doi.org/10.1080/08856257.2016.1254971.

Hillier, A., Goldstein, J., Tornatore, L., Byrne, E., & Johnson, H. M. (2019). Outcomes of a peer mentoring program for university students with disabilities. *Mentoring & Tutoring: Partnership in Learning, 27*(5), 487–508, https://doi.org/10.1080/13611267.2019.1675850.

Hills, M., & Peacock, K. (2022). Replacing power with flexible structure: Implementing flexible deadlines to improve student learning experiences. *Teaching & Learning Inquiry, 10*, https://doi.org/10.20343/teachlearninqu.10.26.

Hinshaw, S. P., & Ellison, K. (2015). *ADHD: What everyone needs to know.* Oxford University Press, Incorporated, https://doi.org/10.1093/wentk/9780190223809.001.0001.

Hitt, S., Sternberg, M., Wadsworth, S., Vaughan, J., Carlson, R., Dansie, E., & Mohrbacher, M. (2015). The higher education landscape for US student service members and veterans in Indiana. *Higher Education (00181560), 70*(3), 535–550, https://doi.org/10.1007/s10734-014-9854-6.

Hoffman, H., Geisthardt, C., & Sucharski, H. (2019). College students and multiple sclerosis: Navigating the college experience. *Journal of Postsecondary Education and Disability, 32*(2), 119–132, https://eric.ed.gov/?id=EJ1228961.

Hoffschmidt, S. J., & Weinstein, C. S. (2003). The influence of silent learning disorders on the lives of women. In M. E. Banks, & E. Kaschak (Eds.), *Women with visible and invisible disabilities: Multiple intersections, multiple issues, multiple therapies* (pp. 81–94). Haworth Press, https://doi.org/10.4324/9781315785875.

Hollins, N., & Foley, A. R. (2013). The experiences of students with learning disabilities in a higher education virtual campus. *Educational Technology Research and Development, 61*(4), 607–624, https://doi.org/10.1007/s11423-013-9302-9.

Hollowell, A., Swartz, J., Myers, E., Erkanli, A., Hu, C., Shin, A., & Bentley-Edwards, K. (2024). Telemedicine services in higher education: A review of college and university websites. *Journal of American College Health, 72*(2), 548–553, https://doi.org/10.1080/07448481.2022.2047703.

Holzberg, D. G., & Ferraro, B. (2021). Speak up: Teaching self-advocacy skills at the communication center to students with disabilities. *Communication Center Journal, 7*(1), 53–72, https://libjournal.uncg.edu/ccj/article/view/2031/pdf.

Hong, B. S. S. (2015). Qualitative analysis of the barriers college students with disabilities experience in higher education. *Journal of College Student Development, 56*(3), 209–226, https://doi.org/10.1353/csd.2015.0032.

Houman, K. M., & Stapley, J. C. (2013). The college experience for students with chronic illness: Implications for academic advising. *NACADA Journal, 33*(1), 61–70, https://doi.org/10.12930/nacada-13-227.

Hubbard, L. E. (2011). *ADHD and comorbid psychiatric disorders: Adult student perspectives on learning needs and academic support* (Publication No. 3602610) [Doctoral dissertation, Lesley University]. ProQuest Dissertations & Theses Global.

Huerta, A. H., & Britton, T. (2022). The nexus of carcerality and access and success in postsecondary education. *American Behavioral Scientist, 66*(10), 1311–1318, https://doi.org/10.1177/00027642211054820.

Hughes, K., Corcoran, T., & Slee, R. (2016). Health-inclusive higher education: Listening to students with disabilities or chronic illnesses. *Higher Education Research and Development, 35*(3), 488–501, https://doi.org/10.1080/07294360.2015.1107885.

Hutson, T. M., McGhee Hassrick, E., Fernandes, S., Walton, J., Bouvier-Weinberg, K., Radcliffe, A., & Allen-Handy, A. (2022). 'I'm just different–that's all–I'm so sorry … ': Black men, ASD and the urgent need for DisCrit Theory in police encounters. *Policing: An International Journal of Police Strategies & Management, 45*(3), 524–537, https://doi.org/10.1108/PIJPSM-10-2021-0149.

Huws, J. C., & Jones, R. S. P. (2015). 'I'm really glad this is developmental': Autism and social comparisons—An interpretative phenomenological analysis. *Autism, 19*(1), 84–90, https://doi.org/10.1177/1362361313512426.

Hux, K., Bush, E., Zickefoose, S., Holmberg, M., Henderson, A., & Simanek, G. (2010). Exploring the study skills and accommodations used by college student survivors of traumatic brain injury. *Brain Injury, 24*(1), 13–26, https://doi.org/10.3109/02699050903446823.

Iniesto, F., Coughlan, T., Lister, K., Devine, P., Freear, N., Greenwood, R., Holmes, W., Kenny, I., McLeod, K., & Tudor, R. (2023). Creating 'a simple conversation': Designing a conversational user interface to improve the experience of accessing support for study. *ACM Transactions on Accessible Computing, 16*(1), 1–29, https://doi.org/10.1145/3568166.

Jack, J. (2014). *Autism and gender: From refrigerator mothers to computer geeks.* University of Illinois Press, https://doi.org/10.5406/illinois/9780252038372.001.0001.

Jackson, A. K. (2023). *Closing the digital divide: Understanding organizational approaches to digital accessibility in higher education* (Publication No. 30485338) [Doctoral dissertation, University of South Dakota]. ProQuest Theses & Dissertations Global.

James, W., Bustamante, C., Lamons, K., Scanlon, E., & Chini, J. J. (2020). Disabling barriers experienced by students with disabilities in postsecondary introductory physics. *Physical Review Physics Education Research, 16*(2), https://doi.org/10.1103/PhysRevPhysEducRes.16.020111.

Jansen, D., Emmers, E., Petry, K., Mattys, L., Noens, I., & Baeyens, D. (2018). Functioning and participation of young adults with ASD in higher education according to the ICF framework. *Journal of Further and Higher Education, 42*(2), 259–275, https://doi.org/10.1080/0309877X.2016.1261091.

Jansen, D., Petry, K., Ceulemans, E., van der Oord, S., Noens, I., & Baeyens, D. (2017). Functioning and participation problems of students with ADHD in higher education: Which reasonable accommodations are effective? *European Journal of Special Needs Education, 32*(1), 35–53, https://doi.org/10.1080/08856257.2016.1254965.

Jones, R. (2021). A phenomenological study of undergraduates with attention deficit hyperactivity disorder and academic library use for research. *New Review of Academic Librarianship, 27*(2), 165–183, https://doi.org/10.1080/13614533.2020.1731560.

Jones, R. E. (2020). *Veterans with PTSD or traumatic brain injury experiences with college and VA and academic services used: A phenomenological study* (Publication No. 28089685) [Doctoral dissertation, Northcentral University]. ProQuest Dissertations & Theses Global.

Kafer, A. (2013). *Feminist, queer, crip.* Indiana University Press.

Kain, S., Chin-Newman, C., & Smith, S. (2019). 'It's all in your head:' Students with psychiatric disability navigating the university environment. *Journal of Postsecondary Education and Disability, 32*(4), 411–425, https://eric.ed.gov/?id=EJ1247131.

Keane, K., & Russell, M. (2014). Using cloud collaboration for writing assignments by students with disabilities: A case study using action research. *Open Praxis, 6*(1), 55–63, https://doi.org/10.5944/openpraxis.6.1.79.

Kearl, B. (2021). Questioning autism's racializing assemblages. *Philosophical Inquiry in Education, 28*(2), 150–162, https://doi.org/10.7202/1082922ar.

Kearns, T. B., & Ruebel, J. B. (2011). Relationship between negative emotion and ADHD among college males and females. *Journal of Postsecondary Education & Disability, 24*(1), 31–42, https://eric.ed.gov/?id=EJ941730.

Kendall-Tackett, K., Marshall, R., & Ness, K. (2003). Chronic pain syndromes and violence against women. In M. E. Banks & E. Kaschak (Eds.), *Women with visible and invisible disabilities: Multiple intersections, multiple issues, multiple therapies* (pp. 45–56). Haworth Press, https://doi.org/10.4324/9781315785875.

Kent, M. (2015). Disability, mental illness, and eLearning: Invisible behind the screen? *The Journal of Interactive Technology & Pedagogy, 8*, 1–18, https://jitp.commons.gc.cuny.edu/disability-mental-illness-and-elearning-invisible-behind-the-screen/.

Kent, M., Ellis, K., & Giles, M. (2018). Students with disabilities and eLearning in Australia: Experiences of accessibility and disclosure at Curtin University. *TechTrends, 62*(6), 654–663, https://doi.org/10.1007/s11528-018-0337-y.

Kercood, S., Lineweaver, T. T., & Kugler, J. (2015). Gender differences in self-reported symptomatology and working memory in college students with ADHD. *Journal of Postsecondary Education & Disability, 28*(1), 41–56, https://eric.ed.gov/?id=EJ1066320.

Kershbaum, S. L., Eisenman, L. T., & Jones, J. M. (2017). *Negotiating disability: Disclosure and higher education.* University of Michigan Press, https://doi.org/10.3998/mpub.9426902.

Kim, J. E., & Zane, N. (2016). Help-seeking intentions among Asian American and white American students in psychological distress: Application of the health belief model. *Cultural Diversity and Ethnic Minority Psychology, 22*(3), 311–321, https://doi.org/10.1037/cdp0000056.

Kimball, E., Vaccaro, A., Tissi-Gassoway, N., Bobot, S. D., Newman, B. M., Moore, A., & Troiano, P. F. (2018). Gender, sexuality, & (dis)ability: Queer perspectives on the experiences of students with disabilities. *Disability Studies Quarterly, 38*(2), 1, https://doi.org/10.18061/dsq.v38i2.5937.

Kinder, J., & Elander, J. (2012). Dyslexia, authorial identity, and approaches to learning and writing: A mixed methods study. *British Journal of Educational Psychology, 82*(2), 289–307, https://doi.org/10.1111/j.2044-8279.2011.02026.x.

King, C. A., Eisenberg, D., Pistorello, J., Coryell, W., Albucher, R. C., Favorite, T., Horwitz, A., Bonar, E. E., Epstein, D., & Zheng, K. (2022). Electronic bridge to mental health for college students: A randomized controlled intervention trial. *Journal of Consulting & Clinical Psychology, 90*(2), 172–183, https://doi.org/10.1037/ccp0000709.

Kirwan, B., & Leather, C. (2011). Students' voices: A report of the student view of dyslexia study skills tuition. *Support for Learning, 26*(1), 33–41, https://doi.org/10.1111/j.1467-9604.2010.01472.x.

Knott, F., & Taylor, A. (2014). Life at university with Asperger syndrome: A comparison of student and staff perspectives. *International Journal of Inclusive Education, 18*(4), 411–426, https://doi.org/10.1080/13603116.2013.781236.

Koch, L. C., Mamiseishvili, K., & Higgins, K. (2014). Persistence to degree completion: A profile of students with psychiatric disabilities in higher education. *Journal of Vocational Rehabilitation, 40*(1), 73–82, https://doi.org/10.3233/JVR-130663.

Kofke, M., & Krazinski, M. (2024, April 11–14). *Weaving DisCrit and neurodiversity studies: A theoretical literature review* [Conference presentation]. AERA 2024 Annual Meeting, Philadelphia, PA, United States, http://tinyurl.com/yrm2cc6w.

Kreider, C. M., Bendixen, R. M., & Lutz, B. J. (2015). Holistic needs of university students with invisible disabilities: A qualitative study. *Physical and Occupational Therapy in Pediatrics, 35*(4), 426–441, https://doi.org/10.3109/01942638.2015.1020407.

Kreider, C. M., Medina, S., Comstock, C. M., Slamka, M. R., Chang-Yu Wu, & Mei-Fang Lan. (2023). Disability-informed graduate-student mentors foster co-regulation for undergraduates in STEM with learning and attention disabilities. *Journal of Postsecondary Education & Disability, 36*(3), 257–275.

Kreiser, N., & White, S. (2015). ASD traits and co-occurring psychopathology: The moderating role of gender. *Journal of Autism & Developmental Disorders, 45*(12), 3932–3938, https://doi.org/10.1007/s10803-015-2580-9.

Krisi, M., & Nagar, R. (2021). The effect of peer mentoring on mentors themselves: A case study of college students. *International Journal of Disability, Development and Education, 70*(5), 803–815, https://doi.org/10.1080/1034912X.2021.1910934.

Kruger, J. S., Godley, S., & Heavey, S. C. (2022). Developing a culture of caring in classrooms: Best practices during a global pandemic and beyond. *Pedagogy in Health Promotion., 8*(2), 99–103, https://doi.org/10.1177/23733799211051403.

Kruger, J. S. (2023). Rethinking penalties for late work: The case for flexibility, equity, and support. *Pedagogy in Health Promotion, 9*(4), 234–236, https://doi.org/10.1177/23733799231198778.

Krumpelman, M. L., & Hord, C. (2021). Experiences of young adults with autism without co-occurring intellectual disability: A review of the literature. *Education and Training in Autism and Developmental Disabilities, 56*(1), 70–82.

Kuder, S. J., & Accardo, A. (2018). What works for college students with autism spectrum disorder. *Journal of Autism and Developmental Disorders, 48*(3), 722–731, https://doi.org/10.1007/s10803-017-3434-4.

Kulshan, T. (2023). *Disabled students' experiences with disability cultural centers and disability culture in U.S. higher education* (Publication No. 30691055) [Doctoral dissertation, City University of Seattle]. ProQuest Dissertations & Theses Global.

Kundu, A. (2019). Understanding college 'burnout' from a social perspective: Reigniting the agency of low-income racial minority strivers towards achievement. *Urban Review, 51*(5), 677–698, https://doi.org/10.1007/s11256-019-00501-w.

Kutscher, E. L., & Tuckwiller, E. D. (2019). Persistence in higher education for students with disabilities: A mixed systematic review. *Journal of Diversity in Higher Education, 12*(2), 136–155, https://doi.org/10.1037/dhe0000088.

Kwon, C., Guadalupe, S. S., Archer, M., & Groomes, D. A. (2023). Understanding career development pathways of college students with disabilities using crip theory and the theory of whole self. *Journal of Diversity in Higher Education, 16*(4), 520–525, https://doi.org/10.1037/dhe0000464.

Kwon, S. J., Kim, Y., & Kwak, Y. (2018). Difficulties faced by university students with self-reported symptoms of attention-deficit hyperactivity disorder: A qualitative study. *Child and Adolescent Psychiatry and Mental Health, 12*(12), https://doi.org/10.1186/s13034-018-0218-3.

Lai, M., Lombardo, M. V., Ruigrok, A. N. V., Chakrabarti, B., Auyeung, B., Szatmari, P., Happé, F., & Baron–Cohen, S. (2017). Quantifying and exploring camouflaging in men and women with autism. *Autism: The International Journal of Research and Practice, 21*(6), 690–702, https://doi.org/10.1177/1362361316671012.

Lambert, D. C., & Dryer, R. (2018). Quality of life of higher education students with learning disability studying online. *International Journal of Disability, Development and Education, 65*(4), 393–407, https://doi.org/10.1080/1034912X.2017.1410876.

Lefler, E. K., Sacchetti, G. M., & Del Carlo, D. I. (2016). ADHD in college: A qualitative analysis. *ADHD Attention Deficit and Hyperactivity Disorders, 8*(2), 79–93, https://doi.org/10.1007/s12402-016-0190-9.

LeGary, R. A., Jr. (2017). College students with autism spectrum disorder: Perceptions of social supports that buffer college-related stress and facilitate academic success. *Journal of Postsecondary Education and Disability, 30*(3), 251–268, https://eric.ed.gov/?id=EJ1163965.

Leopold, A., Rumrill, P., Hendricks, D. J., Nardone, A., Sampson, E., Minton, D., Jacobs, K., Elias, E., & Scherer, M. (2019). A mixed-methodological examination of participant experiences, activities, and outcomes in a technology and employment project for postsecondary students with traumatic brain injuries. *Journal of Vocational Rehabilitation, 50*(1), 3–11, https://doi.org/10.3233/JVR-180983.

Lett, K., Tamaian, A., & Klest, B. (2020). Impact of ableist microaggressions on university students with self-identified disabilities. *Disability and Society, 35*(9), 1441–1456, https://doi.org/10.1080/09687599.2019.1680344.

Levinstein, M. (2018). *A case study of an intrusive advising approach for at-risk, under-prepared and traditionally underrepresented college students* (Publication No. 10985253) [Doctoral dissertation, Kent State University]. ProQuest Dissertations & Theses Global.

Liasidou, A. (2023). Trauma-informed disability politics: Interdisciplinary navigations and implications. *Disability & Society, 38*(4), 683–699, https://doi.org/10.1080/09687599.2021.1946679.

Lightfoot, A., Janemi, R., & Rudman, D. L. (2018). Perspectives of North American postsecondary students with learning disabilities: A scoping review. *Journal of Postsecondary Education and Disability, 31*(1), 57–74, https://eric.ed.gov/?id=EJ1182368.

Linton, S. (1998). *Claiming disability: Knowledge and identity*. New York University Press, https://doi.org/10.18574/nyu/9780814765043.001.0001.

Lipka, O., Forkosh Baruch, A., & Meer, Y. (2019). Academic support model for post-secondary school students with learning disabilities: Student and instructor perceptions. *International Journal of Inclusive Education, 23*(2), 142–157, https://doi.org/10.1080/13603116.2018.1427151.

Lipson, S. K., Kern, A., Eisenberg, D., & Breland-Noble, A. (2018). Mental health disparities among college students of color. *Journal of Adolescent Health, 63*(3), 348–356, https://doi.org/10.1016/j.jadohealth.2018.04.014.

Lister, K., Coughlan, T., Kenny, I., Tudor, R., & Iniesto, F. (2021). Taylor, the disability disclosure virtual assistant: A case study of participatory research with disabled students. *Education Sciences, 11*, https://doi.org/10.3390/educsci11100587.

Lizotte, M. (2018). I am a college graduate: Postsecondary experiences as described by adults with autism spectrum disorders. *International Journal of Education and Practice, 6*(4), 179–191, https://doi.org/10.18488/journal.61.2018.64.179.191.

Lockard, A. J., Hayes, J. A., Neff, K., & Locke, B. D. (2014). Self-compassion among college counseling center clients: An examination of clinical norms and group differences. *Journal of College Counseling, 17*(3), 249–259, https://doi.org/10.1002/j.2161-1882.2014.00061.x.

Lombardi, A., Rifenbark, G. G., Monahan, J., Tarconish, E., & Rhoads, C. (2020). Aided by extant data: The effect of peer mentoring on achievement for college students with disabilities. *Journal of Postsecondary Education and Disability, 33*(2), 143–154.

Losen, D. J., & Orfield, G. (2002). *Racial inequity in special education*. Civil Rights Project, Harvard University.

Lux, S. J. (2016). *The lived experiences of college students with a learning disability and/or attention deficit hyperactivity disorder* (Publication No. 10126486) [Doctoral dissertation, Iowa State University]. ProQuest Dissertations & Theses Global, https://doi.org/10.31274/etd-180810-4637.

MacCullagh, L. (2014). Participation and experiences of students with dyslexia in higher education: A literature review with an Australian focus. *Australian Journal of Learning Difficulties, 19*(2), 93–111, https://doi.org/10.1080/19404 158.2014.921630.

MacCullagh, L., Bosanquet, A., & Badcock, N. A. (2016). University students with dyslexia: A qualitative exploratory study of learning practices, challenges and strategies. *Dyslexia, 23*(1), 3–23, https://doi.org/10.1002/dys.1544.

MacLeod, A., Allan, J., Lewis, A., & Robertson, C. (2018). 'Here I come again': The cost of success for higher education students diagnosed with autism. *International Journal of Inclusive Education, 22*(6), 683–697, https://doi.org/1 0.1080/13603116.2017.1396502.

Madaus, J. W., McKeown, K., Gelbar, N., & Banerjee, M. (2012). The online and blended learning experience: Differences for students with and without learning disabilities and attention deficit/hyperactivity disorder. *International Journal for Research in Learning Disabilities, 1*(1), 21–36, https://eric.ed.gov/?id=EJ1155668.

Madaus, J. W. (2011). The history of disability services in higher education. *New Directions for Higher Education, 2011*(154), 5–15, https://doi.org/10.1002/he.429.

Madaus, J. W., Banerjee, M., Mckeown, K., & Gelbar, N. (2011). Online and blended learning: The advantages and the challenges for students with learning disabilities and attention deficit/hyperactivity disorder. *Learning Disabilities, 17*(2), 69–76, https://eric.ed.gov/?id=EJ961678.

Madaus, J. W., Miller, W. K., & Vance, M. L. (2009). Veterans with disabilities in postsecondary education. *Journal of Postsecondary Education and Disability, 22*(1), 10–17, https://eric.ed.gov/?id=EJ844247.

Mandell, D. S., Ittenbach, R. F., Levy, S. E., & Pinto-Martin, J. (2007). Disparities in diagnoses received prior to a diagnosis of autism spectrum disorder. *Journal of Autism and Developmental Disorders, 37*(9), 1795–1802, https://doi.org/10.1007/s10803-006-0314-8.

Mandell, D. S., Wiggins, L. D., Carpenter, L. A., Daniels, J., DiGuiseppi, C., Durkin, M. S., Giarelli, E., Morrier, M. J., Nicholas, J. S., Pinto-Martin, J., Shattuck, P. T., Thomas, K. C., Yeargin-Allsopp, M., & Kirby, R. S. (2009). Racial/ethnic disparities in the identification of children with autism spectrum disorders. *American Journal of Public Health, 99*(3), 493–498, https://doi.org/10.2105/AJPH.2007.131243.

Mandell, D. S., Listerud, J., Levy, S. E., & Pinto-Martin, J. A. (2002). Race differences in the age at diagnosis among Medicaid-eligible children with autism. *Journal of the American Academy of Child and Adolescent Psychiatry, 41*(12), 1447–1453, https://doi.org/10.1097/00004583-200212000-00016.

Mapes, A. R., & Cavell, T. A. (2023). Students enrolled in a college autism support program: Comparisons with non-enrollees and use of program-sponsored mentoring. *Mentoring & Tutoring: Partnership in Learning, 31*(1), 143–162, https://doi.org/10.1080/13611267.2023.2164990.

Markle, L., Wessel, R. D., & Desmond, J. (2017). Faculty mentorship program for students with disabilities: academic success outcomes (practice brief). *Journal of Postsecondary Education & Disability, 30*(4), 385–392, https://eric.ed.gov/?id=EJ1172790.

Markoulakis, R., & Kirsh, B. (2013). Difficulties for university students with mental health problems: A critical interpretive synthesis. *The Review of Higher Education, 37*(1), 77–100, https://doi.org/10.1353/rhe.2013.0073.

Mason, B. M. (2023). Treating in place: A model of on-campus care for serious mental illnesses. *Journal of College Student Psychotherapy, 37*(3), 227–242, https://doi.org/10.1080/87568225.2021.1961650.

Masuda, A., Anderson, P. L., & Edmonds, J. (2012). Help-seeking attitudes, mental health stigma, and self-concealment among African American college students. *Journal of Black Studies, 43*(7), 773–786, https://doi.org/10.1177/0021934712445806.

Mathew, J., Kraft, S., & Bostwick, J. R. (2021). Opportunities for pharmacists to impact student health on college campuses. *JACCP: Journal of the American College of Clinical Pharmacy, 4*(7), 855–861, https://doi.org/10.1002/jac5.1433.

Maurer-Smolder, C., Hunt, S., & Parker, S. B. (2021). An exploratory study of students with dyslexia in a mixed online and on-campus environment at an Australian regional university. *Australian Journal of Learning Difficulties, 26*(2), 127–151, https://doi.org/10.1080/19404158.2021.1991406.

McConney, A. (2023). Peer helpers at the forefront of mental health promotion at Nelson Mandela University: Insights gained during COVID-19. *Journal of Student Affairs in Africa, 11*(1), 129–144, https://doi.org/10.24085/jsaa.v11i1.4220.

McEwan, R. C., & Downie, R. (2013). College success of students with psychiatric disabilities: Barriers of access and distraction. *Journal of Postsecondary Education and Disability, 26*(3), 233–248, https://eric.ed.gov/?id=EJ1026880.

McGregor, K. K., Langenfeld, N., Van Horne, S., Oleson, J., Anson, M., & Jacobson, W. (2016). The university experiences of students with learning disabilities. *Learning Disabilities Research and Practice, 31*(2), 90–102, https://doi.org/10.1111/ldrp.12102.

McLeod, J. D., Meanwell, E., & Hawbaker, A. (2019). The experiences of college students on the autism spectrum: A comparison to their neurotypical peers. *Journal of Autism and Developmental Disorders, 49*(6), 2320–2336, https://doi.org/10.1007/s10803-019-03910-8.

McSpadden, E. (2022). I'm not crazy or anything: Exploring culture, mental health stigma, and mental health service use among urban community college students. *Community College Journal of Research and Practice, 46*(3), 202–214, https://doi.org/10.1080/10668926.2021.1922321.

Meeks, L. M., Masterson, T. L., & Westlake, G. (2015). Career Connect: A collaborative employment resource model for university students with ASD. *Career Planning and Adult Development Journal, 31*(4), 25–35.

Melara, C. A. (2012). *Factors influencing the academic persistence of college students with ADHD* (Publication No. 3514259) [Doctoral dissertation, University of Southern California]. ProQuest Dissertations & Theses Global.

Menendez, J., Franco, M., Davari, J., Gnilka, P. B., & Ashby, J. S. (2020). Barriers and facilitators to Latinx college students seeking counseling. *Journal of College Student Psychotherapy, 34*(4), 302–315, https://doi.org/10.1080/87568225.2019.1600093.

Meyers, C. A., & Bagnall, R. G. (2015). A case study of an adult learner with ASD and ADHD in an undergraduate online learning environment. *Australasian Journal of Educational Technology, 31*(2), 208–219, https://doi.org/10.14742/ajet.1600.

Michael, R. (2016). The perceived success of tutoring students with learning disabilities: Relations to tutee and tutoring variables. *Journal of Postsecondary Education and Disability, 29*(4), 349–361.

Miller, L. A., Asarta, C. J., & Schmidt, J. R. (2019). Completion deadlines, adaptive learning assignments, and student performance. *Journal of Education for Business., 94*(3), 185–194, https://doi.org/10.1080/08832323.2018.1507988.

Miller, R., Blakeslee, J., & Ison, C. (2020). Exploring college student identity among young people with foster care histories and mental health challenges. *Children and Youth Services Review, 114*, https://doi.org/10.1016/j.childyouth.2020.104992.

Miller, R. A. (2015). 'Sometimes you feel invisible': Performing queer/disabled in the university classroom. *Educational Forum, 79*(4), 377–393, https://doi.org/10.1080/00131725.2015.1068417.

Miller, R. A. (2018). Toward intersectional identity perspectives on disability and LGBTQ identities in higher education. *Journal of College Student Development, 59*(3), 327–346, https://doi.org/10.1353/csd.2018.0030.

Miller, R. A., Dika, S. L., Nguyen, D. J., Woodford, M., & Renn, K. A. (2021). LGBTQ+ college students with disabilities: Demographic profile and perceptions of well-being. *Journal of LGBT Youth, 18*(1), 60–77, https://doi.org/10.1080/19361653.2019.1706686.

Miller, R. A., & Downey, M. (2020). Examining the STEM climate for queer students with disabilities. *Journal of Postsecondary Education and Disability, 33*(2), 169–181, https://eric.ed.gov/?id=EJ1273676.

Miller, R. A., & Smith, A. C. (2021). Microaggressions experienced by LGBTQ students with disabilities. *Journal of Student Affairs Research and Practice, 58*(5), 491–506, https://doi.org/10.1080/19496591.2020.1835669.

Miller, R. A., Wynn, R. D., & Webb, K. W. (2017). Complicating 'coming out': Disclosing disability, gender, and sexuality in higher education. In S. L. Kershbaum, L. T. Eisenman & J. M. Jones (Eds.), *Negotiating disability: Disclosure and higher education* (pp. 115–134). University of Michigan Press, https://doi.org/10.3998/mpub.9426902.

Miller, R. A., Wynn, R. D., & Webb, K. W. (2019). 'This really interesting juggling act': How university students manage disability/queer identity disclosure and visibility. *Journal of Diversity in Higher Education, 12*(4), 307–318, https://doi.org/10.1037/dhe0000083.

Milner, V., McIntosh, H., Colvert, E., & Happé, F. (2019). A qualitative exploration of the female experience of autism spectrum disorder (ASD). *Journal of Autism and Developmental Disorders, 49*(6), 2389–2402, https://doi.org/10.1007/s10803-019-03906-4.

Miodus, S., Allwood, M. A., & Amoh, N. (2021). Childhood ADHD symptoms in relation to trauma exposure and PTSD symptoms among college students: Attending to and accommodating trauma. *Journal of Emotional and Behavioral Disorders, 29*(3), 187–196, https://doi.org/10.1177/1063426620982624.

Miranda, R., Soffer, A., Polanco-Roman, L., Wheeler, A., & Moore, A. (2015). Mental health treatment barriers among racial/ethnic minority versus white young adults 6 months after intake at a college counseling center. *Journal of American College Health, 63*(5), 291–298, https://doi.org/10.1080/07448481.2015.1015024.

Morgan, P. L., Farkas, G., Hillemeier, M. M., & Maczuga, S. (2017). Replicated evidence of racial and ethnic disparities in disability identification in U.S. schools. *Educational Researcher, 46*(6), 305–322, https://doi.org/10.3102/0013189X17726282.

Morgan, P. L., Farkas, G., Hillemeier, M. M., Mattison, R., Maczuga, S., Li, H., & Cook, M. (2015). Minorities are disproportionately underrepresented in special education: Longitudinal evidence across five disability conditions. *Educational Researcher, 44*(5), 278–292, https://doi.org/10.3102/0013189X15591157.

Morgan, P. L., Hillemeier, M. M., Farkas, G., & Maczuga, S. (2014). Racial/ethnic disparities in ADHD diagnosis by kindergarten entry. *Journal of Child Psychology and Psychiatry and Allied Disciplines, 55*(8), 905–913, https://doi.org/10.1111/jcpp.12204.

Morgan, P. L., Staff, J., Hillemeier, M. M., Farkas, G., & Maczuga, S. (2013). Racial and ethnic disparities in ADHD diagnosis from kindergarten to eighth grade. *Pediatrics, 132*(1), 85–93, https://doi.org/10.1542/peds.2012-2390.

Moro, J. (2020). *Against cop shit.* vapor / wear, https://jeffreymoro.com/blog/2020-02-13-against-cop-shit/.

Morris Barr, L. J. (2019). *Person factors affecting student persistence in college reading and writing remediation* (Publication No. 13879269) [Doctoral dissertation, Walden University]. ProQuest Dissertations & Theses Global.

Moss, P., & Dyck, I. (2003). *Women, body, illness: Space and identity in the everyday lives of women with chronic illness.* Rowman & Littlefield Publishers.

Mou, M., & Albagmi, F. M. (2020). Critical discourse analysis of federal and provincial government grants for post-secondary students with disabilities in Alberta and Ontario. *Disability & Society, 38*(7), 1117–1145, https://doi.org/10.1080/09687599.2021.1983418.

Mukherjee, D., Reis, J. P., & Heller, W. (2003). Women living with traumatic brain injury: Social isolation, emotional functioning and implications for psychotherapy. In M. E. Banks, & E. Kaschak (Eds.), *Women with visible and invisible disabilities: Multiple intersections, multiple issues, multiple therapies* (pp. 3–26). Haworth Press, https://doi.org/10.4324/9781315785875.

Mullins, L., & Preyde, M. (2013). The lived experience of students with an invisible disability at a Canadian university. *Disability and Society, 28*(2), 147–160, https://doi.org/10.1080/09687599.2012.752127.

Nachman, B. R. (2020). Enhancing transition programming for college students with autism: A systematic literature review. *Journal of Postsecondary Education and Disability, 33*(1), 81–95, https://eric.ed.gov/?id=EJ1273654.

Nachman, B. R. (2022). 'I need some space–' Autistic community college students and self-advocacy. *Journal of the First-Year Experience & Students in Transition, 34*(2), 9–26, https://www.ingentaconnect.com/contentone/fyesit/fyesit/2022/00000034/00000002/art00001.

National Center for Education Statistics. (2022). *Fast facts: Undergraduate graduation rates.* U.S. Department of Education, Institute of Education Sciences, https://nces.ed.gov/fastfacts/display.asp?id=40.

National Center for Education Statistics. (2023). *Students with disabilities.* U.S. Department of Education, Institute of Education Sciences, https://nces. ed.gov/programs/coe/indicator/cgg/students-with-disabilities.

National Council on Disability. (2019). *Mental health on college campuses: Investments, accommodations needed to address student needs,* https:// www.ncd.gov/report/mental-health-on-college-campuses-investments-accommodations-needed-to-address-student-needs/.

National Institute of Mental Health. (2023a) *Eating disorders.* National Institute of Mental Health (NIMH), https://www.nimh.nih.gov/health/statistics/ eating-disorders.

National Institute of Mental Health. (2023b) *Mental illness.* National Institute of Mental Health (NIMH), https://www.nimh.nih.gov/health/statistics/ mental-illness.

National Technical Assistance Center on Transition, (NTACT). (2019, *Best practices for pre-employment transition services.* National Technical Assistance Center on Transition, https://eric.ed.gov/?q=source%3A%22national+ technical+assistance+center+on+transition%22&ff1=subPlanning&id =ED601230.

Naylor, R., Cox, S., & Cakitaki, B. (2023). Personalised outreach to students on leave of absence to reduce attrition risk. *Australian Educational Researcher, 50*(2), 433–451, https://doi.org/10.1007/s13384-021-00503-2.

Nazaire, M. (2018). *The importance of self-advocacy training for students with disabilities at postsecondary institutions: The disability services officers' perspectives* (Publication No. 10970704) [Doctoral dissertation, La Sierra University]. ProQuest Dissertations & Theses Global.

Nelson, J. M., & Gregg, N. (2012). Depression and anxiety among transitioning adolescents and college students with ADHD, dyslexia, or comorbid ADHD/dyslexia. *Journal of Attention Disorders, 16*(3), 244–254, https://doi. org/10.1177/1087054710385783.

Nelson, J. M., & Harwood, H. (2011). Learning disabilities and anxiety: A meta-analysis. *Journal of Learning Disabilities, 44*(1), 3–17, https://doi. org/10.1177/0022219409359939.

Nelson, L. M., & Reynolds Jr., T. W. (2015). Speech recognition, disability, and college composition. *Journal of Postsecondary Education & Disability, 28*(2), 181–197.

Ness, B. M., Rocke, M. R., Harrist, C. J., & Vroman, K. G. (2014). College and combat trauma: An insider's perspective of the post-secondary education experience shared by service members managing neurobehavioral symptoms. *NeuroRehabilitation, 35*(1), 147–158, https://doi.org/10.3233/ NRE-141098.

Newman, L. A., & Madaus, J. W. (2015). Reported accommodations and supports provided to secondary and postsecondary students with disabilities: National perspective. *Career Development and Transition for Exceptional Individuals, 38*(3), 173–181, https://doi.org/10.1177/2165143413518235.

Newman, L. A., Madaus, J. W., Lalor, A. R., & Javitz, H. S. (2021). Effect of accessing supports on higher education persistence of students with disabilities. *Journal of Diversity in Higher Education, 14*(3), 353–363, https://doi.org/10.1037/dhe0000170.

Nielsen, K. E. (2012). A disability history of the United States. Beacon Press.

Norman, D. A. (2013). The design of everyday things: Revised and expanded edition. Basic Books.

Norris, M. E., & Wood, V. M. (2023). A case study on flexible design: Eliminating documentation requirements for academic adjustments on a test (practice brief). *Journal of Postsecondary Education and Disability, 35*(4), 355–360.

O'Neill, J., Hyun-Ju Kang, Sánchez, J., Muller, V., Aldrich, H., Pfaller, J., & Chan, F. (2015). Effect of college or university training on earnings of people with disabilities: A case control study. *Journal of Vocational Rehabilitation, 43*(2), 93–102, https://doi.org/10.3233/jvr-150759.

Oldfield, J., Rodwell, J., Curry, L., & Marks, G. (2018). Psychological and demographic predictors of undergraduate non-attendance at university lectures and seminars. *Journal of further and Higher Education, 42*(4), 509–523, https://doi.org/10.1080/0309877X.2017.1301404.

Oliver, M. (1983). *Social work with disabled people*. Red Globe Press, https://doi.org/10.1007/978-1-349-86058-6.

Olofsson, Å, Ahl, A., & Taube, K. (2012). Learning and study strategies in university students with dyslexia: Implications for teaching. *Procedia—Social and Behavioral Sciences, 47*, 1184–1193, https://doi.org/10.1016/j.sbspro.2012.06.798.

Orem, S., & Simpkins, N. (2015). Weepy rhetoric, trigger warnings, and the work of making mental illness visible in the writing classroom. *Enculturation: A Journal of Rhetoric, Writing, and Culture*, https://enculturation.net/weepy-rhetoric.

Organization for Autism Research (2018). *Finding your way: A college guide for students on the spectrum*. Organization for Autism Research.

Orr, T. D. (2021). 'Like pushing through slog': Women with depression in online learning. *International Journal of E-Learning & Distance Education, 36*(1), 1–29, https://www.ijede.ca/index.php/jde/article/view/1198.

Oslund, C. (2014). *Supporting college and university students with invisible disabilities: A guide for faculty and staff working with students with autism, AD/HD, language processing disorders, anxiety, and mental illness*. Jessica Kingsley Publishers.

Owens, R. (2020). *Understanding the lived experiences of traumatic brain injury students in online courses* (Publication No. 28090845) [Doctoral dissertation, Walden University]. ProQuest Dissertations & Theses Global, https:// scholarworks.waldenu.edu/dissertations/9215/.

Parker, M. (2023). *A case study: How a top-ranked public institution in Georgia addresses the demand for mental health services* (Publication No. 30691157) [Doctoral dissertation, Baylor University]. ProQuest Dissertations & Theses Global.

Payne, H. (2022). The BodyMind Approach® to support students in higher education: Relationships between student stress, medically unexplained physical symptoms and mental health. *Innovations in Education & Teaching International, 59*(4), 483–494, https://doi.org/10.1080/14703297.2021.18780 52.

Pelka, F. (2012). *What we have done: An oral history of the disability rights movement.* University of Massachusetts Press.

Perlow, E. L., Wells, R. S., Ding, E., Xia, J., MacLean, H., & McCall, A. (2021). Hidden inequality: Financial aid information available to college students with disabilities attending public four-year institutions. *Journal of Student Financial Aid, 50*(3), 1–23, https://doi.org/10.55504/0884-9153.1709.

Pfeifer, M. A., Reiter, E. M., Cordero, J. J., & Stanton, J. D. (2021). Inside and out: Factors that support and hinder the self-advocacy of undergraduates with ADHD and/or specific learning disabilities in STEM. *CBE Life Sciences Education, 20*(2), https://doi.org/10.1187/cbe.20-06-0107.

Phillips, K. G., Nzamubona, K., Houtenville, A. J., O'Neill, J., & Katz, E. E. (2022). Recent college graduates with disabilities: Higher education experiences and transition to employment. *Journal of Postsecondary Education & Disability, 35*(3), 213–228, https://eric.ed.gov/?q=college+preparation&f f1=dtysince_2022&ff2=subOutcomes+of+Education&id=EJ1383752.

Pierce, D. (2022). Out of the shadows: Meeting students' mental health needs takes a community-wide effort. *Community College Journal, 92*(5), 24–31, https://www.aacc.nche.edu/publications-news/ community-college-journal/.

Pingry O'Neill, L. N., Markward, M. J., & French, J. P. (2012). Predictors of graduation among college students with disabilities. *Journal of Postsecondary Education and Disability, 25*(1), 21–36, https://eric.ed.gov/?id=EJ970017.

Pino, & Mortari, L. (2014). The inclusion of students with dyslexia in higher education: A systematic review using narrative synthesis. *Dyslexia, 20*(4), 346–369, https://doi.org/10.1002/dys.1484.

Pionke, J. J. (2017). Toward holistic accessibility: Narratives from functionally diverse patrons. *Reference & User Services Quarterly, 57*(1), 48–56, https:// doi.org/10.5860/rusq.57.1.6442.

Pionke, J. J., Knight-Davis, S., & Brantley, J. S. (2019). Library involvement in an autism support program: A case study. *College and Undergraduate Libraries, 26*(3), 221–233, https://doi.org/10.1080/10691316.2019.1668896.

Pirttimaa, R., Takala, M., & Ladonlahti, T. (2015). Students in higher education with reading and writing difficulties. *Education Inquiry, 6*(1), 5–23, https://doi.org/10.3402/edui.v6.24277.

Poulin, C., & Gouliquer, L. (2003). Part-time disabled lesbian passing on roller blades, or PMS, Prozac, and essentializing women's ailments. In M. E. Banks, & E. Kaschak (Eds.), *Women with visible and invisible disabilities: Multiple intersections, multiple issues, multiple therapies* (pp. 95–108). Haworth Press, https://doi.org/10.4324/9781315785875.

Prevatt, F., Smith, S. M., Diers, S., Marshall, D., Coleman, J., Valler, E., & Miller, N. (2017). ADHD coaching with college students: Exploring the processes involved in motivation and goal completion. *Journal of College Student Psychotherapy, 31*(2), 93–111, https://doi.org/10.1080/87568225.2016.1240597.

Price, M. (2011). *Mad at school: Rhetorics of mental disability and academic life.* University of Michigan Press, https://doi.org/10.3998/mpub.1612837.

Quimby, D., & Agonafer, E. (2023). Culturally matched embedded counseling: Providing empowering services to historically marginalized college students. *Journal of College Student Psychotherapy, 37*(4), 410–430, https://doi.org/10.1080/87568225.2022.2112002.

Ramos-Sánchez, L., & Atkinson, D. R. (2009). The relationships between Mexican American acculturation, cultural values, gender, and help-seeking intentions. *Journal of Counseling & Development, 87*(1), 62–71, https://doi.org/10.1002/j.1556-6678.2009.tb00550.x.

Randolph, T. S. (2012). *Students with disabilities' experience and description of integrating into an academic community in higher education: A phenomenological study* (Publication No. 3498407) [Doctoral dissertation, Capella University]. ProQuest Dissertations & Theses Global.

Ravert, R. D., Russell, L. T., & O'Guin, M. B. (2017). Managing chronic conditions in college: Findings from prompted health incidents diaries. *Journal of American College Health, 65*(3), 217–222, https://doi.org/10.1080/07448481.2016.1266640.

Raye, L. (2017). Soft toys as instructional technology in higher education: The case of Llewelyn the Lynx. *Journal of Effective Teaching, 17*(1), 35–51.

Reader, C. M. (2018). *The effectiveness of intrusive advising programs on academic achievement and retention in higher education* (Publication No. 10792407) [Doctoral dissertation, Indiana State University]. ProQuest Dissertations & Theses Global.

Redpath, J., Kearney, P., Nicholl, P., Mulvenna, M., Wallace, J., & Martin, S. (2013). A qualitative study of the lived experiences of disabled post-transition students in higher education institutions in Northern Ireland. *Studies in Higher Education, 38*(9), 1334–1350, https://doi.org/10.10 80/03075079.2011.622746.

Retherford, K. S., & Schreiber, L. R. (2015). Camp campus: College preparation for adolescents and young adults with high-functioning autism, Asperger syndrome, and other social communication disorders. *Topics in Language Disorders, 35*(4), 362–385, https://doi.org/10.1097/TLD.0000000000000070.

Reynolds, E. M. (2022). *Leading through the integration of university health and counseling centers* (Publication No. 30521795) [Doctoral dissertation, Johnson & Wales University]. ProQuest Dissertations & Theses Global, https://scholarsarchive.jwu.edu/dissertations/AAI30521795.

Richardson, G. (2021). Dyslexia in higher education. *Educational Research and Reviews, 16*(4), 125–135, https://doi.org/10.5897/err2021.4128.

Richman, E. L., Rademacher, K. N., & Maitland, T. L. (2014). Coaching and college success. *Journal of Postsecondary Education & Disability, 27*(1), 33–52.

Rith–Najarian, L., Gong-Guy, E., Flournoy, J. C., & Chavira, D. A. (2024). Randomized controlled trial of a web-based program for preventing anxiety and depression in university students. *Journal of Consulting & Clinical Psychology, 92*(1), 1–15, https://doi.org/10.1037/ccp0000843.

Roberts, A. L., Gilman, S. E., Breslau, J., Breslau, N., & Koenen, K. C. (2011). Race/ethnic differences in exposure to traumatic events, development of post-traumatic stress disorder, and treatment-seeking for post-traumatic stress disorder in the United States. *Psychological Medicine, 41*(1), 71–83, https://doi.org/10.1017/S0033291710000401.

Roberts, J. B., Crittenden, L. A., & Crittenden, J. C. (2011). Students with disabilities and online learning: A cross-institutional study of perceived satisfaction with accessibility compliance and services. *Internet and Higher Education, 14*(4), 242–250, https://doi.org/10.1016/j.iheduc.2011.05.004.

Roberts, N., & Birmingham, E. (2017). Mentoring university students with ASD: A mentee-centered approach. *Journal of Autism & Developmental Disorders, 47*(4), 1038–1050, https://doi.org/10.1007/s10803-016-2997-9.

Robinson H., Al-Freih M., Kilgore T. A., Kilgore W. (2023). Critical pedagogy and care ethics: Feedback as care. In Köseoğlu S., Veletsianos G., Rowell C. (Eds.), *Critical Digital Pedagogy in Higher Education* (pp. 31–45). Athabasca University Press, https://doi.org/10.15215/aupress/9781778290015.003.

Rolander, K., Severson-Irby, E., & Massey, H. (2021). Inclusive virtual instruction: A case study of a bridge program for adult learners who have disabilities. *COABE Journal: The Resource for Adult Education, 10*(2), 96–108.

Rothwell, C. A., & Shields, J. J. (2021). Setting students up for success: Academic skills before and after participation in 2–4–8, a proactive advising model for students with disabilities. *Journal of Postsecondary Education and Disability, 34*(4), 349–359, https://eric.ed.gov/?id=EJ1342747.

Russell, G. (2020). Critiques of the neurodiversity movement. In S. K. Kapp (Ed.), *Autistic community and the neurodiversity movement: Stories from the frontline* (pp. 287–303). Palgrave Macmillan, https://doi.org/10.1007/978-981-13-8437-0_21.

Russell, M. L., & Pearl, D. (2020). Virtual self-advocacy training development for freshmen students with a documented learning difference (practice brief). *Journal of Postsecondary Education and Disability, 33*(2), 201–206, https://eric.ed.gov/?id=EJ1273700.

Rutherford, E. N. (2013). *An exploration of support factors available to higher education students with high functioning autism or Asperger syndrome* (Publication No. 3606486) [Doctoral dissertation, Lamar University—Beaumont]. ProQuest Dissertations & Theses Global.

Saia, T. (2022). Disability cultural centers in higher education: A shift beyond compliance to disability culture and disability identity. *Journal of Postsecondary Education & Disability, 35*(1), 17–30.

Salzer, M. S. (2012). A comparative study of campus experiences of college students with mental illnesses versus a general college sample. *Journal of American College Health, 60*(1), 1–7, https://doi.org/10.1080/07448481.2011.552537.

Samlan, H., Shetty, A., & McWhirter, E. H. (2021). Gender and racial-ethnic differences in treatment barriers among college students with suicidal ideation. *Journal of College Student Psychotherapy, 35*(3), 272–289, https://doi.org/10.1080/87568225.2020.1734133.

Samuels, E. (2003). My body, my closet: Invisible disability and the limits of coming-out discourse. *GLQ, 9*(1–2), 233–255, https://doi.org/10.1215/10642684-9-1-2-233.

Sarrett, J. C. (2018). Autism and accommodations in higher education: Insights from the autism community. *Journal of Autism and Developmental Disorders, 48*(3), 679–693, https://doi.org/10.1007/s10803-017-3353-4.

Saviet, M., & Ahmann, E. (2021). ADHD coaches' experiences with and perceptions of between-session communication with clients: A focus group. *Coaching: An International Journal of Theory, Research & Practice, 14*(2), 127–141, https://doi.org/10.1080/17521882.2021.1877754.

Savvidou, G., & Loizides, F. (2016). *Investigating commercially available technology for language learners in higher education within the high functioning disability spectrum.* [Conference presentation]. EUROCALL: Conference on Computer-Assisted Language Learning, Limassol, Cyprus, https://eric.ed.gov/?id=ED572197.

Sayman, D. M. (2015). I still need my security teddy bear: Experiences of an individual with autism spectrum disorder in higher education. *The Learning Assistance Review, 20*(1), 77–98, https://eric.ed.gov/?id=EJ1058012.

Schaffer, G. (2013). Assessing compensatory strategies and motivational factors in high-achieving postsecondary students with attention deficit/hyperactivity disorder. *Journal of Postsecondary Education and Disability, 26*(1), 89–99, https://eric.ed.gov/?id=EJ1026827.

Scheef, A. R., McKnight-Lizotte, M., & Gwartney, L. (2019). Supports and resources valued by autistic students enrolled in postsecondary education. *Autism in Adulthood, 1*(3), 219–226, https://doi.org/10.1089/aut.2019.0010.

Schepman, S., Weyandt, L., Schlect, S. D., & Swentosky, A. (2012). The relationship between ADHD symptomology and decision making. *Journal of Attention Disorders, 16*(1), 3–12, https://doi.org/10.1177/1087054710372496.

Schindler, V. P., & Kientz, M. (2013). Supports and barriers to higher education and employment for individuals diagnosed with mental illness. *Journal of Vocational Rehabilitation, 39*(1), 29–41, https://doi.org/10.3233/JVR-130640.

Schneps, M. H., Chen, C., Pomplun, M., Wang, J., Crosby, A. D., & Kent, K. (2019). Pushing the speed of assistive technologies for reading. *Mind, Brain, and Education, 13*(1), 14–29, https://doi.org/10.1111/mbe.12180.

Schreier, B. A., Anderson, C. L., Galligan, P. K., Greenbaum, B., Corkery, J., Schnelle, T., Gates, C., Hong, J. E., & Kivlighan III, D. M. (2023). Embedded therapists: Who do they serve? How are they funded? And where are they housed? A foundational survey of emerging models. *Journal of College Student Psychotherapy, 37*(2), 144–154, https://doi.org/10.1080/87568225.2021.1913686.

Schwenk, H. T., Lightdale, J. R., Arnold, J. H., Goldmann, D. A., & Weitzman, E. R. (2014). Coping with college and inflammatory bowel disease: Implications for clinical guidance and support. *Inflammatory Bowel Diseases, 20*(9), 1618–1627, https://doi.org/10.1097/MIB.0000000000000124.

Scotch, R. K. (1988). Disability as the basis for a social movement: Advocacy and the politics of definition. *Journal of Social Issues, 44*(1), 159–172, https://doi.org/10.1111/j.1540-4560.1988.tb02055.x.

Seale, J. (2017). From the voice of a 'socratic gadfly': A call for more academic activism in the researching of disability in postsecondary education. *European Journal of Special Needs Education, 32*(1), 153–169, https://doi.org/10.1080/08856257.2016.1254967.

Seale, J., Colwell, C., Coughlan, T., Heiman, T., Kaspi-Tsahor, D., & Olenik-Shemesh, D. (2021). 'Dreaming in colour': Disabled higher education students' perspectives on improving design practices that would enable them to benefit from their use of technologies. *Education and Information Technologies, 26*(2), 1687–1719, https://doi.org/10.1007/s10639-020-10329-7.

Seehuus, M., Moeller, R. W., & Peisch, V. (2021). Gender effects on mental health symptoms and treatment in college students. *Journal of American*

College Health, 69(1), 95–102, https://doi.org/10.1080/07448481.2019.16562 17.

Seng, J. S., Lopez, W. D., Sperlich, M., Hamama, L., & Reed Meldrum, C. D. (2012). Marginalized identities, discrimination burden, and mental health: Empirical exploration of an interpersonal-level approach to modeling intersectionality. *Social Science & Medicine, 75*(12), 2437–2445, https://doi.org/10.1016/j.socscimed.2012.09.023.

Serry, T., Oates, J., Ennals, P., Venville, A., Williams, A., Fossey, E., & Steel, G. (2018). Managing reading and related literacy difficulties: University students' perspectives. *Australian Journal of Learning Difficulties, 23*(1), 5–30, https://doi.org/10.1080/19404158.2017.1341422.

Shapiro, J. P. (1994). No pity: People with disabilities forging a new civil rights movement (1st ed.). Times Books.

Sharma, A. K. (2022). Use of assistive technologies for inclusive education in Visva-Bharati Library Network. *Library Progress (International), 42*(1), 231–236, https://doi.org/10.5958/2320-317X.2022.00025.3.

Shea, L. C., Hecker, L., & Lalor, A. R. (2018). *From disability to diversity: College success for students with learning disabilities, ADHD, and autism spectrum disorder*. National Resource Center for The First Year Experience & Students in Transition.

Shipherd, J. C., Lynch, K., Gatsby, E., Hinds, Z., DuVall, S. L., & Livingston, N. A. (2021). Estimating prevalence of PTSD among veterans with minoritized sexual orientations using electronic health record data. *Journal of Consulting & Clinical Psychology, 89*(10), 856–868, https://doi.org/10.1037/ccp0000691.

Shmulsky, S., & Gobbo, K. (2019). Autism support in a community college setting: Ideas from intersectionality. *Community College Journal of Research and Practice, 43*(9), 648–652, https://doi.org/10.1080/10668926.2018.152227 8.

Siebers, T. A. (2016). *Disability theory*. University of Michigan Press, https://doi.org/10.3998/mpub.309723.

Siko, L. (2018). *Wearable technology for self-monitoring of academic engagement in college students with autism spectrum disorder* (Publication No. 10814889) [Doctoral dissertation, George Mason University]. ProQuest Dissertations & Theses Global.

Silberman, S. (2015). *Neurotribes: The legacy of autism and the future of neurodiversity*. Avery.

Sinclair, J. (2013). Why I dislike 'person first' language. *Autonomy, 1*(2), https://blogs.exeter.ac.uk/exploringdiagnosis/files/2017/03/Sinclair-Why-I-Dislike-First-Person-Language.pdf.

Slaughter, S. (2014). Retheorizing academic capitalism: Actors, mechanisms, fields, and networks. In B. Cantwell, & I. Kauppinen (Eds.), *Academic capitalism in the age of globalization* (pp. 10–32). Johns Hopkins University Press, https://doi.org/10.1353/book.49259.

Slaughter, S., & Leslie, L. L. (1997). *Academic capitalism: Politics, policies, and the entrepreneurial university.* Johns Hopkins University Press, https://doi.org/10.56021/9780801855498.

Slaughter, S., & Rhoades, G. (2004). *Academic capitalism and the new economy: Markets, state, and higher education.* Johns Hopkins University Press, https://doi.org/10.56021/9780801879494.

Smith, C. F. (2017). *Advanced undergraduate students with dyslexia: Perceptions of social supports that buffer college-related stress and facilitate academic success* (Publication No. 10686714) [Doctoral dissertation, Southern Connecticut State University]. ProQuest Dissertations & Theses Global.

Sokal, L., & Desjardins, N. (2016). What students want you to know: Promoting achievement in postsecondary students with anxiety disorders. *Journal on Excellence in College Teaching, 27*(3), 111–136.

Soni, A. (2017). Students' experiences of academic success with dyslexia: A call for alternative intervention. *Support for Learning, 32*(4), 387–405, https://doi.org/10.1111/1467-9604.12182.

Sontag-Padilla, L., Williams, D., Kosiewicz, H., Daugherty, L., Kane, H., Gripshover, S., & Miller, T. (2023). *How community colleges can support student mental health needs.* Research Brief. RB-A2552-1, https://doi.org/10.7249/RBA2552-1.

Spencer, G., Lewis, S., & Reid, M. (2018). Living with a chronic health condition: Students' health narratives and negotiations of (ill) health at university. *Health Education Journal, 77*(6), 631–643, https://doi.org/10.1177/0017896917738120.

Stampoltzis, A., Tsitsou, E., Plesti, H., & Kalouri, R. (2015). The learning experiences of students with dyslexia in a Greek higher education institution. *International Journal of Special Education, 30*(2), 157–170, https://internationalsped.com/ijse/issue/view/16.

Stanger, S. B., & Lucas, S. J. (2024). Using indirect service-learning to promote evidence-based digital mental health tools on college campuses. *Teaching of Psychology, 51*(2), 240–247, https://doi.org/10.1177/00986283221084005.

Stapleton, L., & James, L. (2020). Not another all-white study: Challenging color-evasiveness ideology in disability scholarship. *Journal of Postsecondary Education and Disability, 33*(3), 215–222.

Stark, M. D., Ayala, C., Quinn, B. P., Guerra-Stella, L., Gomez, J., & Cunningham, L. (2023). Solution-focused mentoring with college students diagnosed with a learning disability. *Journal of Postsecondary Education & Disability, 36*(3), 225–240.

Stein, K. F. (2013). DSS and accommodations in higher education: Perceptions of students with psychological disabilities. *Journal of Postsecondary Education and Disability, 26*(2), 145–161, https://eric.ed.gov/?id=EJ1026925.

Stewart, R. (2023). *'Nothing about us without us': A qualitative inquiry of disabled student activists creating disability cultural centers on college campuses* (Publication No. 30489361) [Doctoral dissertation, California State University, Sacramento]. ProQuest Dissertations & Theses Global.

Strnadová, I., Hájková, V., & Květoňová, L. (2015). Voices of university students with disabilities: Inclusive education on the tertiary level—A reality or a distant dream? *International Journal of Inclusive Education, 19*(10), 1080–1095, https://doi.org/10.1080/13603116.2015.1037868.

Suciu, M. (2014). UNE Mentoring Program for Students Living with Autism Spectrum Disorders (ASDs). *Journal of the Australian & New Zealand Student Services Association, (44)*, 55–59.

Sullivan, P., Blacker, M., & Murphy, J. (2019). Levels of psychological distress of Canadian university student-athletes. *Canadian Journal of Higher Education, 49*(1), 47–59, https://doi.org/10.47678/cjhe.v49i1.188192.

Tanabe, K. O., Hayden, M. E., Zunder, B., & Holstege, C. P. (2023). Identifying vulnerable populations at a university during the COVID-19 pandemic. *Journal of American College Health, 71*(1), 14–17, https://doi.org/10.1080/074 48481.2021.1877142.

Tarallo, A. E. (2012). *Understanding students with autism spectrum disorders in higher education* (Publication No. 3525797) [Doctoral dissertation, Northeastern University]. ProQuest Dissertations & Theses Global.

Taylor, M., Turnbull, Y., Bleasdale, J., Francis, H., & Forsyth, H. (2016). Transforming support for students with disabilities in UK higher education. *Support for Learning, 31*(4), 367–384, https://doi. org/10.1111/1467-9604.12143.

Taylor, Z. W. (2020). Clicking in the dark: Are student financial aid websites accessible for students with disabilities? *Journal of Student Financial Aid, 49*(2), 1–17, https://doi.org/10.55504/0884-9153.1687.

Terras, K. (2020). Comparing disability accommodations in online courses: A cross-classification. *Journal of Educators Online, 17*(2), https://www.thejeo. com/archive/2020_17_2/terras_anderson_grave.

Thomas, M., Rostain, A., & Prevatt, F. A. (2013). ADHD diagnosis and treatment in young adults and college students. In A. Joffee (Ed.), *Adolescent medicine: State of the art reviews*. American Academy of Pediatrics.

Thomas, N. G. (2020). Using intrusive advising to improve student outcomes in developmental college courses. *Journal of College Student Retention: Research, Theory & Practice, 22*(2), 251–272, https://doi. org/10.1177/1521025117736740.

Thompson, C., Falkmer, T., Evans, K., Bölte, S., & Girdler, S. (2018). A realist evaluation of peer mentoring support for university students with autism. *British Journal of Special Education, 45*(4), 412–434, https://doi.org/10.1111/1467-8578.12241.

Thompson, L. S. (2021). The dyslexic student's experience of education. *South African Journal of Higher Education, 35*(6), 204–221, https://doi.org/10.20853/35-6-4337.

Thomson, E. A. (2022). *Exploring the impact of a disability cultural center on disabled students in higher education* (Publication No. 29330572) [Doctoral dissertation, University of Illinois at Chicago]. ProQuest Dissertations & Theses Global.

Timmerman, L. C., & Mulvihill, T. M. (2015). Accommodations in the college setting: The perspectives of students living with disabilities. *The Qualitative Report, 20*(10), 1609–1626, https://doi.org/10.46743/2160-3715/2015.2334.

Tlili, A., Altinay, Z., Aydin, C. H., Huang, R., & Sharma, R. C. (2022). Reflections on massive open online courses (MOOCS) during the COVID-19 pandemic: A bibliometric mapping analysis. *Turkish Online Journal of Distance Education, 23*(3), 1–17, https://doi.org/10.17718/tojde.1137107.

Tobin, T. J., & Behling, K. (2018). *Reach everyone, teach everyone: Universal design for learning in higher education.* West Virginia University Press.

Toft, A., Franklin, A., & Langley, E. (2019). Young disabled and LGBT+: Negotiating identity. *Journal of LGBT Youth, 16*(2), 157–172, https://doi.org/10.1080/19361653.2018.1544532.

Toller, L., & Farrimond, H. (2021). The unpredictable body, identity, and disclosure: Identifying the strategies of chronically ill students at university. *Disability Studies Quarterly, 41*(2), https://doi.org/10.18061/dsq.v41i2.7049.

Tomas, M., Rostain, A., & Prevatt, F. A. (2013). ADHD diagnosis and treatment in young adults and college students. In A. Joffee (Ed.), *Adolescent medicine: State of the art reviews.* American Academy of Pediatrics, https://doi.org/10.1542/9781581108736-adhd_diagnosis.

Toor, N., Hanley, T., & Hebron, J. (2016). The facilitators, obstacles and needs of individuals with autism spectrum conditions accessing further and higher education: A systematic review. *Journal of Psychologists and Counsellors in Schools, 26*(2), 166–190, https://doi.org/10.1017/jgc.2016.21.

Tops, W., Glatz, T., Premchand, A., Callens, M., & Brysbaert, M. (2020). Study strategies of first-year undergraduates with and without dyslexia and the effect of gender. *European Journal of Special Needs Education, 35*(3), 398–413, https://doi.org/10.1080/08856257.2019.1703580.

Townsend, T. G., Kaltman, S., Saleem, F., Coker-Appiah, D., & Green, B. L. (2020). Ethnic disparities in trauma-related mental illness: Is ethnic identity a buffer? *Journal of Interpersonal Violence, 35*(11), 2164–2188, https://doi.org/10.1177/0886260517701454.

Tran, A. G. T. T. (2022). Race/ethnicity and stigma in relation to unmet mental health needs among student-athletes. *Journal of College Student Psychotherapy, 36*(4), 392–409, https://doi.org/10.1080/87568225.2021.1881 859.

Trevisan, D. A., Leach, S., Iarocci, G., & Birmingham, E. (2021). Evaluation of a peer mentorship program for autistic college students. *Autism in Adulthood: Challenges and Management, 3*(2), 187–194, https://doi.org/10.1089/ aut.2019.0087.

Turosak, A., & Siwierka, J. (2021). Mental health and stigma on campus: Insights from students' lived experience. *Journal of Prevention and Intervention in the Community, 49*(3), 266–281, https://doi.org/10.1080/1085 2352.2019.1654264.

Urban Institute (n.d.). *Time to degree.* Retrieved from https:// collegeaffordability.urban.org/covering-expenses/time-to-degree/#/.

Vaccaro, A., Lee, M. N., Tissi-Gassoway, N., Kimball, E. W., & Newman, B. M. (2020). Gender and ability oppressions shaping the lives of college students: An intracategorical, intersectional analysis. *Journal of Women and Gender in Higher Education, 13*(2), 119–137, https://doi.org/10.1080/263791 12.2020.1780134.

Van Hees, V., Moyson, T., & Roeyers, H. (2015). Higher education experiences of students with autism spectrum disorder: Challenges, benefits and support needs. *Journal of Autism and Developmental Disorders, 45*(6), 1673–1688, https://doi.org/10.1007/s10803-014-2324-2.

VanderLind, R. (2018). *Identity development, stigma, and academic resilience in college students with mental illness* (Publication No. 10985622) [Doctoral dissertation, Texas State University—San Marcos]. ProQuest Dissertations & Theses Global, https://digital.library.txstate.edu/handle/10877/7369.

Varkula, L. C., Beauchemin, J. D., Facemire, S. D., & Bucher, E. C. (2017). Differences between students with and without disabilities in college counseling. *Journal of Postsecondary Education and Disability, 30*(2), 173–184, https://eric.ed.gov/?id=EJ1153557.

Venville, A., Mealings, M., Ennals, P., Oates, J., Fossey, E., Douglas, J., & Bigby, C. (2016). Supporting students with invisible disabilities: A scoping review of postsecondary education for students with mental illness or an acquired brain injury. *International Journal of Disability, Development and Education, 63*(6), 571–592, https://doi.org/10.1080/1034912X.2016.1153050.

Venville, A., & Street, A. F. (2014). Hearing voices: Qualitative research with postsecondary students experiencing mental illness. *International Journal of Training Research, 12*(1), 45–56, https://doi.org/10.5172/ijtr.2014.12.1.45.

Verduce, C. (2019, *Ideas for creating a career center and disability services office collaboration.* National Association of Colleges and Employers (NACE) Individuals with Disabilities Affinity Impact Team. Retrieved May 1, 2024, from https://community.naceweb.org/blogs/cindy-verduce1/2019/10/08/ideas-for-creating-a-career-center-and-disability.

Vincent, J., Potts, M., Fletcher, D., Hodges, S., Howells, J., Mitchell, A., Mallon, B., & Ledger, T. (2017). 'I think autism is like running on Windows while everyone else is a Mac': Using a participatory action research approach with students on the autistic spectrum to rearticulate autism and the lived experience of university. *Educational Action Research, 25*(2), 300–315, https://doi.org/10.1080/09650792.2016.1153978.

Walker, N. (2021). *Neuroqueer heresies: Notes on the neurodiversity paradigm, autistic empowerment, and postnormal possibilities* (1st ed.). Autonomous Press.

Ward, D., & Webster, A. (2018). Understanding the lived experiences of university students with autism spectrum disorder (ASD): A phenomenological study. *International Journal of Disability, Development and Education, 65*(4), 373–392, https://doi.org/10.1080/1034912X.2017.1403573.

Wei, X., Christiano, E., Yu, J., Blackorby, J., Shattuck, P., & Newman, L. (2014). Postsecondary pathways and persistence for STEM versus non-STEM majors: Among college students with an autism spectrum disorder. *Journal of Autism & Developmental Disorders, 44*(5), 1159–1167, https://doi.org/10.1007/s10803-013-1978-5.

Wei, X., Yu, J., Shattuck, P., McCracken, M., & Blackorby, J. (2013). Science, technology, engineering, and mathematics (STEM) participation among college students with an autism spectrum disorder. *Journal of Autism & Developmental Disorders, 43*(7), 1539–1546, https://doi.org/10.1007/s10803-012-1700-z.

Weimer, M. (2013). *Learner-centered teaching: Five key changes to practice* (2nd ed.). Jossey-Bass.

Wendell, S. (2001). Unhealthy disabled: Treating chronic illnesses as disabilities. *Hypatia, 16*(4), 17–33, https://doi.org/10.1111/j.1527-2001.2001.tb00751.x.

Wennås Brante, E. (2013). 'I don't know what it is to be able to read': How students with dyslexia experience their reading impairment. *Support for Learning, 28*(2), 79–86, https://doi.org/10.1111/1467-9604.12022.

Whillans, A., & West, C. (2022). Alleviating time poverty among the working poor: A pre-registered longitudinal field experiment. *Scientific Reports, 12*(719), https://doi.org/10.1038/s41598-021-04352-y.

White, G. W., Summers, J. A., Zhang, E., & Renault, V. (2014). Evaluating the effects of a self-advocacy training program for undergraduates with disabilities. *Journal of Postsecondary Education & Disability, 27*(3), 229–244, https://eric.ed.gov/?id=EJ1048818.

White, S. W., Elias, R., Salinas, C. E., Capriola, N., Conner, C. M., Asselin, S. B., Miyazaki, Y., Mazefsky, C. A., Howlin, P., & Getzel, E. E. (2016). Students with autism spectrum disorder in college: Results from a preliminary mixed methods needs analysis. *Research in Developmental Disabilities, 56,* 29–40, https://doi.org/10.1016/j.ridd.2016.05.010.

Williams, D. A. (2015). *Understanding the experiences of adult students with brain injuries in online learning* (Publication No. 3687981) [Doctoral dissertation, Capella University]. ProQuest Dissertations & Theses Global.

Wilson, M. (2012). Stories of resilience: Learning from adult students' experiences of studying with dyslexia in tertiary education. *Journal of Adult Learning Aotearoa New Zealand, 40*(1), 110–126.

Winberg, K., Bertilsdotter Rosqvist, H., & Rosenberg, D. (2019). Inclusive spaces in post-secondary education: Exploring the experience of educational supports for people with a neuropsychiatric disability. *International Journal of Inclusive Education, 23*(12), 1263–1276, https://doi.org/10.1080/13603116.2018.1445303.

Winter, J. A. (2003). The development of the disability rights movement as a social problem solver. *Disability Studies Quarterly, 23*(1), 33–61, https://doi.org/10.18061/dsq.v23i1.399.

Wiorkowski, F. (2015). The experiences of students with autism spectrum disorders in college: A heuristic exploration. *Qualitative Report, 20*(6), 847–863, https://doi.org/10.46743/2160-3715/2015.2163.

Wissa, U. A., & Avdic, A. (2017). Flexible study pace, mental disabilities and e-learning: Perceived problems and opportunities. *Proceedings of the European Conference on E-Learning (ECEL),* 527–534.

Withington, K., & Schroeder, H. L. (2017). Rolling with the semester: An assignment deadline system for improving student outcomes and regaining control of the workflow. *Journal of Student Success and Retention, 4*(1), 1–31, https://www.jossr.org/wp-content/uploads/2017/10/Rolling-with-the-semester-Final.pdf.

Wladis, C., Hachey, A. C., & Conway, K. M. (2024). It's about time, part II: Does time poverty contribute to inequitable college outcomes by gender and race/ethnicity? *AERA Open, 10,* https://doi.org/10.1177/23328584241237971.

Woof, V. G., Hames, C., Speer, S., & Cohen, D. L. (2021). A qualitative exploration of the unique barriers, challenges and experiences encountered by undergraduate psychology students with mental health problems. *Studies in Higher Education, 46*(4), 750–762, https://doi.org/10.1080/03075079.2019.1652809.

Woolf, E., & de Bie, A. d. (2022). Politicizing self-advocacy: Disabled students navigating ableist expectations in postsecondary education. *Disability Studies Quarterly, 42*(1), https://doi.org/10.18061/dsq.v42i1.8062.

Wright, S. A. (2011). *Functional impairments of college students with attention deficit/ hyperactivity disorder and necessary modifications for higher education* (Publication No. 3476515) [Doctoral dissertation, West Virginia University]. ProQuest Dissertations & Theses Global, https://doi.org/10.33915/etd.3043.

Wu, I., & Molina, R. M. (2019). Self-determination of college students with learning and attention challenges. *Journal of Postsecondary Education & Disability, 32*(4), 359–375, https://eric.ed.gov/?id=EJ1247134.

Yamamoto, K. K., & Black, R. S. (2015). Standing behind and listening to native Hawaiian students in the transition process. *Career Development and Transition for Exceptional Individuals, 38*(1), 50–60, https://doi.org/10.1177/2165143413498412.

Young, E. W. D. (2012). *Understanding the psycho-social and cultural factors that influence the experience of attention-deficit/hyperactivity disorder (ADHD) in Chinese American college students: A systems approach* (Publication No. 3513866) [Doctoral dissertation, University of Southern California]. ProQuest Dissertations & Theses Global.

Zafran, H., Tallant, B., & Gelinas, I. (2011). A first-person exploration of the experience of academic reintegration after first episode psychosis. *International Journal of Psychosocial Rehabilitation, 16*(1), 27–43.

Zeedyk, S. M., Bolourian, Y., & Blacher, J. (2019). University life with ASD: Faculty knowledge and student needs. *Autism, 23*(3), 726–736, https://doi.org/10.1177/1362361318774148.

Zilvinskis, J., Barber, R. E., Brozinsky, J. L., & Hochberg, S. R. (2020). Measuring the differential effects of behaviors of academic advisors for students with disabilities. *NACADA Journal, 40*(2), 15–32, https://doi.org/10.12930/NACADA-19-25.

Zilvinskis, J., Barber, R. E., Brozinsky, J. L., Hochberg, S. R., & Weston, M. (2023). Mediation effects of academic advising behaviors for first-year students with learning disabilities and mental health disorders. *Journal of Postsecondary Education and Disability, 35*(4), 319–337.

Zinzow, H., Amstadter, A., McCauley, J., Ruggiero, K., Resnick, H., & Kilpatrick, D. (2011). Self-rated health in relation to rape and mental health disorders in a national sample of college women. *Journal of American College Health, 59*(7), 588–594, https://doi.org/10.1080/07448481.2010.520175.

Index

About the Team

Alessandra Tosi was the managing editor for this book.

Lucy Barnes proof-read this manuscript. Annie Hine compiled the index.

Jeevanjot Kaur Nagpal designed the cover. The cover was produced in InDesign using the Fontin font.

Cameron Craig typeset the book in InDesign and produced the paperback and hardback editions. The main text font is Tex Gyre Pagella and the heading font is Californian FB.

Cameron also produced the PDF and HTML editions. The conversion was performed with open-source software and other tools freely available on our GitHub page at https://github.com/OpenBookPublishers.

Jeremy Bowman created the EPUB.

Raegan Allen was in charge of marketing.

This book was peer-reviewed by an anonymous referee. Expert in their fields, our readers give their time freely to help ensure the academic rigour of our books. We are grateful for their generous and invaluable contributions

This book need not end here...

Share

All our books — including the one you have just read — are free to access online so that students, researchers and members of the public who can't afford a printed edition will have access to the same ideas. This title will be accessed online by hundreds of readers each month across the globe: why not share the link so that someone you know is one of them?

This book and additional content is available at
https://doi.org/10.11647/OBP.0420

Donate

Open Book Publishers is an award-winning, scholar-led, not-for-profit press making knowledge freely available one book at a time. We don't charge authors to publish with us: instead, our work is supported by our library members and by donations from people who believe that research shouldn't be locked behind paywalls.

Join the effort to free knowledge by supporting us at
https://www.openbookpublishers.com/support-us

We invite you to connect with us on our socials!

BLUESKY	MASTODON	LINKEDIN
@openbookpublish .bsky.social	@OpenBookPublish @hcommons.social	open-book-publishers

Read more at the Open Book Publishers Blog
https://blogs.openbookpublishers.com

You may also be interested in:

Higher Education for Good
Teaching and Learning Futures
Laura Czerniewicz and Catherine Cronin (Eds)

https://doi.org/10.11647/obp.0363

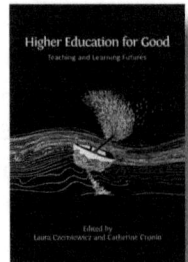

Dire Straits-Education Reforms
Ideology, Vested Interests and Evidence
Montserrat Gomendio and José Ignacio Wert

https://doi.org/10.11647/obp.0332

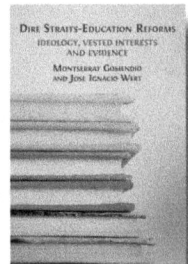

Like Nobody's Business
An Insider's Guide to How US University Finances Really Work
Andrew C. Comrie

https://doi.org/10.11647/obp.0240

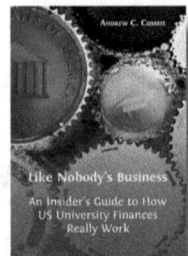

Milton Keynes UK
Ingram Content Group UK Ltd.
UKHW022154111124
451073UK00008B/296

9 781805 113751